SEXUALITY
ALL THAT MATTERS

Biography

Louise Foxcroft is a historian, writer and broadcaster who specializes in medical perceptions of the human body and at the way these influence our present-day experience. Her doctorate was from the University of Cambridge and her books include *The Making of Addiction: The use and abuse of opiates in nineteenth-century Britain* (Ashgate, 2007), *Hot Flushes, Cold Science: A history of the modern menopause* (Granta, 2009) which won the Longman/*History Today* Book of the Year award, and *Calories & Corsets: A history of dieting over 2,000 years* (Profile Books, 2011). She has written for *The Times, Independent, Guardian, London Review of Books* and other publications, has appeared on BBC TV and Radio and was told a saucy joke in an interview with Sir David Frost on Al Jazeera English.

Louise was a Non-Alcoholic Trustee on the General Service Board of Alcoholics Anonymous (GB) for five years, speaking to national and international conferences, and to MPs, policy-makers and professional agencies at Westminster, the Welsh National Assembly and the Scottish Parliament. She is company director of Village Underground in Shoreditch, London (www.villageunderground.co.uk).

SEXUALITY

Louise Foxcroft

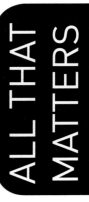

ALL THAT MATTERS

First published in Great Britain in 2014 by Hodder and Stoughton. An Hachette UK company.

This edition published 2014.

British Library Cataloguing in Publication Data: a catalogue record for this title is available from the British Library.

ISBN: 9781444798609

eISBN: 9781444798616

10 9 8 7 6 5 4 3 2

2015

The publisher has used its best endeavours to ensure that any website addresses referred to in this book are correct and active at the time of going to press. However, the publisher and the author have no responsibility for the websites and can make no guarantee that a site will remain live or that the content will remain relevant, decent or appropriate.

The publisher has made every effort to mark as such all words which it believes to be trademarks. The publisher should also like to make it clear that the presence of a word in the book, whether marked or unmarked, in no way affects its legal status as a trademark.

Every reasonable effort has been made by the publisher to trace the copyright holders of material in this book. Any errors or omissions should be notified in writing to the publisher, who will endeavour to rectify the situation for any reprints and future editions.

Cover image ©

Typeset by Cenveo® Publisher Services.

Printed and bound in Great Britain by CPI Group (UK) Ltd., Croydon, CR0 4YY.

John Murray Learning policy is to use papers that are natural, renewable and recyclable products and made from wood grown in sustainable forests. The logging and manufacturing processes are expected to conform to the environmental regulations of the country of origin.

John Murray Learning

338 Euston Road

London NW1 3BH

www.hodder.co.uk

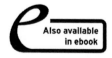

Also available in ebook

Contents

1 What does sexuality mean?   1

2 The start of sexuality   9

3 Celebration and punishment   21

4 Savagery and tenderness   43

5 Sexuality meets science   55

6 Truth and sexuality   73

7 Sexuality and identity   85

8 New anxieties   105

9 Sexuality is as wide as the sea   117

100 Ideas   130

Sources and Further Reading   140

Acknowledgements   144

Index   145

1

What does sexuality mean?

What freedom men and women could have, were they not constantly tricked and trapped and enslaved and tortured by their sexuality! The only drawback in that freedom is that without it one would not be a human. One would be a monster

John Steinbeck, East of Eden *(1952)*

Sexuality is innate, inescapable. It is a sometimes marvellous, sometimes monstrous, mosaic that has evolved over the centuries. Every generation thinks it has invented sexuality and so it has, because sexuality is not a given but a constantly changing network of interlinked ideas, knowledge, desires, pleasures, controls and exploitation. Forget any notion of sexuality as homogeneous, either in experience or understanding, despite the many attempts made to persuade or coerce people into a 'safe' or coherent mould. Sexuality is potentially disruptive.

According to the OED, sexuality is the quality and expression of being sexual, having a sexual nature, instinct, or feelings. Most people are pretty sure they know what 'sexuality' means but the concept is fundamentally ambiguous and multi-faceted: we now include heterosexuality, asexuality, homosexuality, hypersexuality, paraphilias, asphyxiophilia, pomosexuality, pansexuality, and so many others that it risks turning this short book into merely a very long list. Sexuality is seen as a question of biology, or an urge; it is applied to individuals and groups, to behaviours, styles, and expression – but how does it exist beyond the word? Perhaps it is best understood as a chaotic social construct. In most societies sex is, and has been, a private act, and so the definitions, boundaries and 'rules' have become quite specific. This being so, the sanctions, especially those applied to relatively powerless groups or populations, have been hijacked to bolster arguments about morality, politics, and science; a great deal of academic study on sexuality has an agenda, too, explicit or not. Any appraisal of sexuality must involve an understanding of difference, of what the shifting target of 'normal' means, of secrecy and knowledge, of who should know, say or do what, and to whom. It is an enormous, difficult and obviously fascinating task, and there has never been any shortage of those willing to try: who, as has been asked, could make the bedroom a laboratory?

Marquis de Sade The 120 Days of Sodom (1785):

Your narrations must be decorated with the most numerous and searching details; the precise way and extent to which we may judge how the passion which you describe relates to human manners and man's character is determined by your willingness to disguise no circumstance; and what is more, the least circumstance is apt to have an immense influence upon the procuring of that kind of sensory irritation we expect from your stories.

'Sexuality' is an eighteenth-century European term and, according to the French philosopher Michel Foucault, its use marked the development of fields of knowledge, rules and norms. Sexuality now seemed to be knowable through regulatory systems of power – religious, judicial, medical and scientific – and the term gave people a body of thought through which they could see themselves. This great change, wrote Foucault in his influential *The History of Sexuality* (1979), was a new interpretation of desire. He tells our own 'story' back to us as one in which we believe ourselves to have been more liberal in our sexual attitudes, behaviours and language in the past, but have somehow lost this freedom and tolerance. Then, during the nineteenth century, a repressive regime emerged that made sex taboo, tried to confine it within the boundaries of marriage, and silenced us. The State began to organize sexuality and to dictate what was acceptable and unacceptable through specialized knowledge; illicit sexualities were expressed in 'other' places such as asylums and brothels. But, as Foucault points out, there was actually a 'discursive explosion'. Everyone was discussing and analysing sexuality – and, even today, we continue to talk endlessly, and hypocritically, about sexual silence. This may appear to be a process of control, but it is actually 'the very production of sexuality' because it has as much to do with our imaginations and desires, in variation or deviation, as it does with physiological sex. In 1905, Freud was arguing that the expression of sexuality could also be found in apparently non-sexual activities, especially in artistic creation and intellectual enquiry. Take, for example, the potent Greek myth of Leda and the Swan – the rape of Leda by Zeus in the form of a swan caused her to give birth to her babies in eggs. This has been portrayed and analysed by so many in so many ways, from Michelangelo to Fernando Botero, from Rubén Darío to Lou Reed.

W. B. Yeats, *Leda and the Swan* (1924):

A sudden blow: the great wings beating still

Above the staggering girl, her thighs caressed

By the dark webs, her nape caught in his bill,

He holds her helpless breast upon his breast.

How can those terrified vague fingers push

The feathered glory from her loosening thighs?

And how can body, laid in that white rush,

But feel the strange heart beating where it lies?

A shudder in the loins engenders there

The broken wall, the burning roof and tower

And Agamemnon dead.

Being so caught up,

So mastered by the brute blood of the air,

Did she put on his knowledge with his power

Before the indifferent beak could let her drop?

The vast sex-scape of experience and response over time drips with humour and anxiety, proscription,

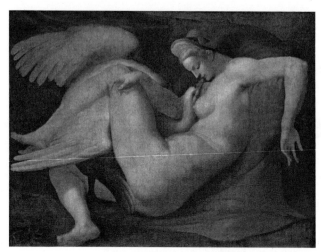

▲ 'Leda and the Swan', Peter Paul Rubens, c.1598–60

prescription, polemic and wit – none of which are as far apart as they seem, or as some might like them to be. As Giovanni Sinibaldi, the Pope's physician writing on sex in the seventeenth century, asked, does 'the same road lead to torment and to delight?'.

This introductory book looks at sexuality from antiquity to the twenty-first century, exploring expression, changing attitudes, and regulation. It looks at bodies of authorized and unauthorized sexual knowledge from scientific, religious, medical, philosophical, and political ideas to letters, diaries, court cases, and medical histories that reveal popular assumptions and individual experiences. Sexuality is where the personal and public collide, and prejudice too: as Samuel Johnson wrote in 1763, 'Nature has given women so much power, that law has wisely given them little'.

The greater sexualization of our society has undoubtedly muddied people's expectations and understanding, and is at risk of turning sexuality into a looks-and-performance-oriented, one-trick-pony parody, when it is a much deeper and more complicated creature. Asking questions about sexuality, about identity and behaviour and how far we have been defined by these concepts throughout history, reminds us of how complex we are. This makes for a more compassionate understanding of people in the past and their idiosyncrasies, as well as of our own today. So what did earlier commentators think they were writing about and why? What was their purpose? How different was their understanding of sexuality to our more recent ideas?

2

The start of sexuality

It is by the power of names, of signs originally arbitrary and insignificant, that the course of the imagination has in great measure been guided

Jeremy Bentham

The oldest handbooks on sex are Chinese, the earliest dating from c.2000 BCE. Three sexological works were found among fourteen Taoist medical manuscripts in a tomb in Hunan province in 1973. In these writings, sexual satisfaction was deemed paramount because of the mystical benefits, good health and pleasures it bestowed, as long as it was enjoyed according to certain theories that didn't undermine individuals and society. Sex, 'the play of the clouds and the rain', was a sacred duty for men and women. It was seen as part of a natural order (sex and nature share the same word, 'xing'), and outdoor sex was considered the most satisfying, with each tree and flower suggesting a different position. The particular practices and philosophies, voluntarily accepted, attempted to define potentially problematic sexuality, because procreation, property, disease, and death were much closer bedfellows then than they are now. There was no link between eroticism and sin.

Men were advised to have sex with as many women as possible, but they should always be sparing with their *qi* (energy) – writings suggest that they 'Love one hundred times without emission' – and should replenish it with female *yin*, meaning that it was important for her to orgasm, too. Female masturbation was considered to be commonplace, inevitable and good. Under the same theory, so was lesbianism, which was known as *Mojingzi*, 'rubbing mirrors' or 'mirror grinding'. Male homosexuality was discussed in the oldest texts, and catamites – young men who served as sexual partners to adult homosexuals and bisexuals – originated during the reign of the mythical Yellow Emperor, who became immortal after congress with 12,000 women, c.4,000 years ago. These texts and their erotic illustrations were titillating but they also gave advice and information and were often prescriptive, showing that sexuality has always been about more than physiology.

Prescribed sexual knowledge has always been open to subversion: Neo-Confucianist puritans later tried to ban Taoist ideas because of their perceived threat to male hegemony. Many of these 'books on the art of the bedroom' were destroyed, though some fragments survive, including: *The Secret Instructions of the Jade Chamber* (Yufangmijue); Sun Simiao's *Essential Prescriptions Worth a Thousand Pieces of Gold* (Qianjin yaofang); and *Exposition of Cultivating the True Essence by the Great Immortal of the Purple Gold Splendour* (Zijin guangyao daxian xiuzhen yanyi). During the first century CE, Buddhism arrived in China via the Silk Road, and it challenged the prevalent ideas on sexuality. For Buddhists, sexuality was part of suffering – people could be enslaved by their desires, especially sexual desire, which was considered to be the strongest form – but the Chinese thought this hypocritical and portrayed it negatively in art and literature. Joseph Needham, a twentieth-century scientist, historian and sinologist, was 'profoundly convinced' that the Chinese were more enlightened with their 'most perfect combination of the rational and the romantic' and that Christian thinking, for example, was greatly mistaken in separating 'love carnall' and 'love seraphick'. Taoist ideas on sexuality, he believed, lead to greater acceptance and contentment, and to a better world with less cruelty and greed.

In India, the Sanskrit text, *Kama Sūtra of Vatsyayana*, pulled together works as much as 3,000 years old and, in its present form, was collated in around the second century CE. *'Kama'* is erotic desire and *'Sūtra'* is the thread that holds everything together. It is a guide to gracious living with advice on sex and sexual behaviours, including games, marriage, family life, choosing a lover, different embraces, and courtesans. Homosexuality is discussed as the 'third nature' and should 'be engaged in and enjoyed for its own sake as one of the arts', but only for some castes. Ancient texts also included hermaphroditism; it appears in the Vedas, Hindu and Jain texts, which formulated sexual categories as early as the sixth century BCE, and is referred to in Plato's *Banquet* where Aristophanes says:

Anciently the nature of mankind was not the same as now, but different. For at first there were three sexes of human beings, not two only, namely male and female, as at present, but a third besides, common to both the others – of which the name remains, though the sex itself has vanished. For the androgynous sex then existed, both male and female; but now it only exists as a name of reproach.

Kama Sūtra of Vatsyayana

Chapter IX, trans. Richard Burton (1883): The male servants of some men carry on the mouth congress with their masters. It is also practised by some citizens, who know each other well, among themselves. Some women of the harem, when they are amorous, do the acts of the mouth on the yonis of one another, and some men do the same thing with women ... When a man and woman lie down in an inverted order, i.e. with the head of the one towards the feet of the other and carry on this congress, it is called the "congress of a crow". For the sake of such things courtesans abandon men possessed of good qualities, liberal and clever, and become attached to low persons, such as slaves and elephant drivers. The Auparishtaka, or mouth congress, should never be done by a learned Brahman, by a minister that carries on the business of a state, or by a man of good reputation, because though the practice is allowed by the Shastras, there is no reason why it should be carried on, and need only be practised in particular cases ... after all, these things being done secretly, and the mind of the man being fickle, how can it be known what any person will do at any particular time and for any particular purpose.

Early erotica emphasizes the mores of different times and cultures. Ovid's erotodidactic poem, *Ars Amatoria*, is some 2,000 years old, and begins with the seductive encouragement, 'Should anyone here not know the art of love, read this, and learn by reading how to love'. Though an ancient poem describing an ancient culture, it can be read by the modern reader as directly relevant: sexuality remains a preoccupying experience central to humanity. *Ars Amatoria* was witty and controversial, and many of its conventions and warnings persist, not least the idea of conquest. Ovid advised men to use any trick to win a woman, for 'every woman alive, the plainest included/ feels she's a loveable beauty/But often a pretender begins to love for real/often, he becomes what he made out to be'. His advice to women was not to 'drink more than your head will stand ... It's a horrible thing to see a woman really drunk. When she's in that state, she deserves to be had by the first comer ... A sleeping woman is a whoreson temptation to a man to transgress the bounds of modesty'. Debates over appropriate sexual behaviours seem to continue largely unchanged.

The Emperor Augustus, in a case of early literary censorship, banished Ovid from Rome for writing his 'poetry as sex' (and for an unknown act of folly). Ovid himself had defended his work by saying that he wrote it in fun, that love could not be immoral; but, centuries later in fifteenth-century Florence, his works were cast into the great bonfire of Savonarola as being erotic, impious, and corrupting. It did not stop there: Christopher Marlowe's translation was banned in 1599; in 1895 a Victorian critic declared that it was 'perhaps the most immoral poem ever written'; in 1910 it was 'calculated to undermine the social fabric'; in 1924 it was denounced as 'a shameless compendium of profligacy'; and a copy was seized by US Customs in 1930 for glorifying extra-marital sex, and undermining marriage and stability.

The Roman historian Suetonius (c.69 – after 122 CE) revealed the lives of the Roman Empire's first leaders in *The Twelve Caesars*. Tiberius collected 'Bevies of girls and young men ... as adepts in unnatural practices, and known as *spinitrae*, [who] would copulate before him in groups of three, to excite his waning passions. A number of small rooms were furnished with the most indecent pictures and statuary possible, also certain erotic manuals from Elephantis in Egypt; the inmates of the establishment would know exactly what was expected of them' (orgies have never gone out of fashion – in 1966 Malcolm Muggeridge remarked that, 'An orgy looks particularly alluring seen through the mists of righteous indignation'). Tiberius was an orgiastic voyeur, one of many. The Emperor Heliogabalus presided over an orgy which ended in death; the sated participants slowly smothered by rose petals released from ceiling nets while he watched – which was all he could do as he had been castrated by his physician attempting to create a vagina for him.

Ribald sexuality was familiar to the Romans; it served to instruct, amuse, warn, and excite. The infamous marble sculpture of Pan and a she-goat in sexual congress raises many questions in the viewer. For example, are humans closer to divine godliness or to base animality? What does it mean to be male or female, and what are their relations to one another? The sculpture was discovered in 1752 and kept in a restricted collection in the cellars of the royal palace at Portici on the Bay of Naples, but it soon became notorious. Various art historians came to see the sculpture, even though some thought it so obscene it should be tossed into a volcano. Johann Joachim Winckelmann visited the sculpture several times between 1758 and 1767, but didn't want to be known as the first to apply for a viewing licence for such a piece of pornography. In the nineteenth century it was moved to a reserved gallery in what is now the National Archaeological Museum of Naples and was kept hidden until 2000; now it is a major piece on show in public exhibitions. In ancient Herculaneum and Pompeii, erotic art was ubiquitous: sculptures, graffiti, tintinnabula (phallic wind-chimes) hanging from doorways, sex scenes on everything from drinking cups to oil lamps, and dining rooms and bath-houses were decorated with wall-paintings of people engaged in such activities as cunnilingus or with multiple partners. Images meant different things in different contexts: they might be humorous, aggressive, sacred, secular, obscene or seductive; they might be exquisitely or crudely executed. They reflected the reality of everyday life and what people did in private, rather than society's moralistic rules of sexuality, which could be condemnatory when it came to, for example, oral sex.

Many of the instructional texts were written by elite, educated men for one another, but were also expected to filter through into a wider society. In classical Greek and Roman thought, men and women were almost different species, defined by their sex rather than their sexuality: in classical humoral theory, males were thought of as warm and dry, females as cold and damp. Their respective roles and freedoms in society reflected their differences, usually to the detriment of the female sex (this idea was tenacious: Samuel Haworth's *Anthropologia* (1680), among others, states that females were 'procreated by accident out of a weaker seede' and were 'nothing else

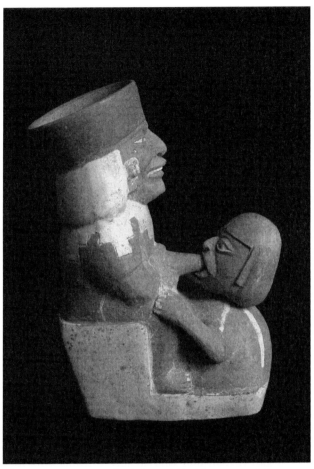

▲ 'Mochica Pottery with Erotic Scene', Mochica pottery dating
from the first to eighth century AD at the Museo de Arqueologia,
Antropologia e Historia in Trujillo, Peru
© *Atlantide Phototravel/Corbis.*

but an error or aberration of Nature'). The influential physician Galen (d.200 BCE) held that male and female genitalia were homologous, i.e. they have similar position, structure and function, and this is known as the 'one-sex model'. He describes female sexual organs as a sort of substandard, interior version of the male's, they correspond to his but are not turned outwards due to lack of heat; at moments of great physical activity it was thought possible that a woman might change gender by pushing her organs out and becoming a man. The hierarchical one-sex model didn't work in the opposite direction, however, as the male body was considered the ideal, far superior to the inherently pathological female. It was immensely influential and wasn't seriously opposed until the prominent, sixteenth-century French physician, André Du Laurens, reinterpreted Galen's ideas. He shared the Platonist view that eroticism was a source of insanity and could plunge its victim into animality and uncontrollable passions, robbing the human soul of divine light and reason. Concupiscence was to be feared but it could be treated, and Du Laurens believed that love had its own physiology: the image of the object of desire goes from the eyes to the liver; the liver then called upon the heart and these two major organs mounted an attack upon reason leading to a bout of *melanckolie amoureuse*. Love, then, was hellish, bestial and mad, capable of corrupting the individual and society at large. This was medicine with moral muscle from the start.

Plato (d.347 BCE), Greek philosopher and student of Socrates, considered sexual desire (Eros) in the *Ladder of Love – The Ascent to Beauty Itself* (*Symposium*). The

Priestess Diotima argues with Socrates that, since we desire what we do not have, and Eros desires the good and the beautiful, then Eros – sexual desire – must lack both beauty and goodness. But, she cries, 'must that be foul which is not fair?'. The Ladder of Love is a route upwards that gives us power and hope over base sexuality. Love of a beautiful body is at the bottom rung; but if you love one beautiful body then you must love them all, leading to the discovery that the beauties of the body are nothing compared to spiritual loveliness even if it is within an unlovely body. This love leads to a more noble nature and to the beauty of laws and institutions, and then to the realization that all beauty is like another and that the beautiful body is not so momentous. The beauty of learning and knowledge is the final revelation at the top of the ladder, the 'very soul of beauty'. And when you have understood that, you are safe. Heavenly beauty itself, 'unsullied, unalloyed, and freed from the mortal taint that haunts the frailer loveliness of flesh and blood' came from this, where:

you will never be seduced again by the charm of gold, of dress, of comely boys, or lads just ripening to manhood; you will care nothing for the beauties that used to take your breath away and kindle such a longing in you.

Ideas and assumptions about sexuality have also been encapsulated in mythology, as useful, popular stories explaining difficult and wild ideas. Myths are heavy with tradition, being exotic, familiar, dramatic, exploratory and often subversive. They allow mortals to step into the lives of gods, to see a man's love for his wife's sister, a daughter's fear of her mother: the gods were astonishingly promiscuous in their sex lives, emotionally and physically fierce, and could take different shapes, viz. Leda and the Swan. Zeus, the 'Father of Gods and men', in the form of an eagle, also abducted Ganymede to serve as a cup-bearer in Olympus – this story is a mythologization of the Greek penchant for pederasty, the socially acceptable erotic relationship between men and youths. Ganymede was the only one of Zeus's lovers who was granted immortality, and he personifies beautiful young men who are the object of homosexual desire and love. Myths allow us to change ourselves, at least in our imagination, and to question sexual identity: Tiresias, in Greek mythology a blind Theban seer, was changed from man to woman by the Goddess Hera, who later argued with her husband, Zeus, whether women experienced less sexual pleasure. Having experienced both, Tiresias told her that women had ten times the pleasure of men. That debate, of who has the more pleasure, has historically occupied the musings of philosophers and physicians, as well as most men and women. Camille Paglia, social critic and 'dissident feminist', wrote of mythical stereotypes that they are 'the West's stunning sexual personae ... the moment there is imagination, there is myth'. Myth and sexuality still coexist today, not always happily.

3

Celebration and punishment

People can die of mere imagination

Geoffrey Chaucer

Emergent Christian dogmas brought sin and sex together. After the Fall of Man and the release of carnal consciousness, the lapsarian world was prey to this forbidden knowledge; erotica was unfit for modest eyes and ears. What Foucault called a 'technology of the flesh' had begun to shift then current ideas about human sexuality. The lyrical Old Testament 'Song of Songs' vied with the Manichean idea of the body as the cause of evil and Augustine of Hippo's 'Lust's darkness'. (Saint Augustine's *Confessions* were written c.397 BCE). Augustine had been forced to marry a ten-year-old girl, which powerfully affected his thoughts about sexuality. Sex seemed to be a culpable act of woe, and his ideas on original sin continue to wield immense influence on the present day, especially with regard to women and how they are negatively perceived as inherently 'bad' among some groups.

Ecclesiastes 7:26 (King James Bible, 1611)

And I finde more bitter then death, the woman whose heart is snares & nets, and her handes as bands: who so pleaseth God, shall escape from her, but the sinner shall be taken by her.

Augustinian ideology spread serendipitously as monks went into exile, taking his ideas with them from North

Africa into the monastic world of Europe, and ideas of temptation, sin and punishment became increasingly vehement. Yet some sexual knowledge was allowed, for the begetting of children, for example, and conjugal consolation, but the Church tried to harness sexuality in an attempt to protect the innocent and vulnerable from lust, lewdness and corruption. It was a bit of a balancing act between the necessary conjugal sex and the filth of fornication. Certain sexual acts were fine, others were not; it wasn't that church dogma ruled against all sex acts but it was in the business of proscribing certain kinds of non-procreative sex. The Quran, too, forbade homosexuality, sodomy, fornication, and sex during menstruation, while emphasizing the good of legitimate, hygienic intimacy between husband and wife – after sex they should wash and pray. Religion and law were often interchangeable: by the thirteenth century, for example, English law determined that sodomites be buried alive.

Medieval and early modern Europe experienced a period of enormous social change, pestilence, rising nationalism, conflict, rebellion and renaissance. Within this turbulence, sexuality was both constrained and crudely celebrated, for example in the twelfth-century scatological poem, where lovers Turgibus and Rainberge plight their troth in a coprophiliac way:

La Chanson d'Audigier

To the noble lord she turned and bent down

And showed him her arse and cunt, all she had got.

"Come on forward, said she, my young lord's son,

Squat down by me, and let's shit together.

Last night I ate an abundance of plums,

And now my arse is a gutter that runs,

And I didn't bring any rag with me.

You have a beautiful scarlet surcoat,

Wipe round my arse for me with your coat-tails,

Or else you won't have the gift of my love...

Then he wiped all round her arse for her.

Whereupon, squatting, they plighted their troth.

This is a good point at which to say that erotica is to do with sexual sharing whereas pornography is sexual using, and, as much as Turgibus and Rainberge shared their erotic betrothal, negative views of the 'nature' of female sexuality were – and are – still rife. Its allegedly all-consuming corruption is a common and frightening fallacy that has biblical authority in the Book of Proverbs, Chapter 30. In the epistolary tale of Abelard and Heloise, she writes to her illicit lover:

What misery for me – born as I was to be the cause of such a crime! Is it the general lot of women to bring total ruin on great men? Hence the warning about women in Proverbs:

'... do not let your heart entice you into her ways, do not stray down her paths; she has wounded and laid low so many, and the strongest have all been her victims. Her house is the way to hell, and leads down to the halls of death'.

Such ideas were occasionally challenged, though, by writers such as Christine de Pizan (1365–1430), who produced some of the earliest 'feminist' works. She was educated, which was a rare thing for women then. When widowed, she became the first European woman to support herself and her family through her writing. Her most important books, *The Book of the City of Ladies* (1404-05) and *Book of the Treasury of Ladies* (1405), placed women on the same level as men. Sex and sexuality were not decisive when it came to worth: 'neither the loftiness nor the lowliness of a person lies in the body according to the sex, but in the perfection of conduct and virtues'. She also attacked the double standards of her day by asking, 'if women are so flighty, fickle, changeable, susceptible, and inconstant ... why is it that their suitors have to resort to such trickery to have their way with them? And why don't women quickly succumb to them, without the need for all this skill and ingenuity in conquering them?'

Boccaccio's *The Decameron*, written in the fourteenth century, similarly attacked state and church corruption, and placed sexuality back within the natural order of things (it had a wide influence, from Shakespeare to George Eliot). *The Decameron* comprises a hundred tales of sex and death told over ten nights by ten young men and women during a devastating plague time, and it defies conventional mores. Likewise, Chaucer's *Canterbury Tales*, of which more than eighty sixteenth-century copies survive and reveal its popularity, is a collection of pilgrims' stories written between 1387 and 1400, which give voice to various characters with humour, bawdiness, and reflective morality.

'The concupiscence of the flesh' in the arts has long been a cause of sexual gratification, a source of visual guidance and a reason for denunciation. During this time, Europe's great artists were making images of sexuality for private and public viewing and for themselves. Leonardo da Vinci (1452–1519) believed images were superior to words when it came to arousing the senses: one of his patrons had asked him to mask out the religious iconography in a painting of the Madonna because it made him feel both lustful and ashamed. Theologians attempted to police sexual behaviours through the Catholic confessional and Protestant Church court prosecutions – moral and medical regulation of sexuality and erotic identities have stretched from the fifteenth century to the present day, linking sin and pathology with devastating and guilt-inducing effect.

Fear and rationality overlapped – arguably they still do across many cultures – and sexuality was mired in medicine, magic and misogyny. The lustful desires of women were a major cause of anxiety, which found one outlet through witch-hunts: the *Malleus Maleficarum* ('The Hammer of Witches'), written by a German Catholic clergyman in 1487, railed against female sexuality, saying that 'all witchcraft comes from carnal lust, which is in women insatiable'. Images from that time – for example, woodcuts of witches kissing the Devil's arse – can be as titillating, shaming and shocking today, as, presumably, they were to people then. The invention of the printing press in the mid-fifteenth century meant that texts and images of sex and sexuality became increasingly available and popular in the Western world.

In the East, coeval with this, cultural ideals of sexuality conveyed a celebratory power of sex and love; a different take on Eros. Hindus were positive about sexuality and the freedoms of eroticism. Homosexuality and lesbianism, '*swayamvara*' (self-chosen), had appeared in an eleventh-century Sanskrit story cycle, *Kathasaritsagara*; some explicitly sexual Urdu poems in the *rekhti* genre use '*dogana*', a term of address between female lovers, as well as '*chapti*' which means rubbing or clinging. The fourteenth-century Bengali epic poem, *Krittivasa Ramayana*, discusses a child born of sex between two women, taken from an ancient medical text, *Sushruta Samhita*, but says that such a child would be born without bones. And the fifteenth-century Tunisian work, *The Perfumed Garden of Sensual Delight* by Muhammad ibn Muhammad al-Nafzawi, offered lavish advice on behaviours and techniques, as well as remedies for sexual diseases. Translations didn't appear in Europe, however, until the middle of the nineteenth century when it was brought across by the French Army from its occupation in North Africa.

> *For if every one of our affections*
> *displeases heaven,*
> *To what purpose would God have*
> *made the world?*

A heady erudition suffused the European Renaissance and allowed the publication of Giovanni Benedetto Sinibaldi's Greek-titled *Geneanthropeia*, the first standard Western work on sexuality. The English, however, made do with a bowdlerized edition, *Rare Verities, the Cabinet of Venus Unlock'd*, in 1658, which reached a wider audience. In it, the literary elite were told that sex had marvellous and 'Salubrious effects', but only if 'rendered lawful by matrimony and free of sin [lest] the sinner lose his soul if not his health'. The book was part of a growing medical discourse on sexuality and was entertaining, anatomical and regulatory. As such it has been called 'pornodidascalian', meaning a work that mixes forbidden instruction and illicit pleasure, and is educational as well as pornographically entertaining – these works could not succeed *nisi pruriant*, without arousing the reader. The term 'pornography' didn't appear until

1857, in an English medical dictionary defined as 'a description of prostitutes or of prostitution, as a matter of public hygiene'; however, by 1864 it was being defined in the way we would understand it today. Sinibaldi's book discussed deviant practices and extreme sex lives, welcomed aphrodisiacs but not boys as lust-objects, and noted that flagellation was a complete prodigy for how could it be 'that pleasure comes from pain, sweet from bitter, lust from bloody wounds?'. The author enjoyed libidinous folklore and salacious anecdotes, revelled in the concupiscence of women, included a section on the thousand 'figurae' possible in intercourse, and even pondered whether nature could 'more opportunely have located the male organ elsewhere, and why did she endow him with one only, and not two?'.

Women were regarded by medicine as being little more than their reproductive systems, hence they were possessed of less ability to reason than men and, so therefore, in need of control. Reinier de Graaf, known as the first modern reproductive biologist, wrote

> *There are three things which are insatiable – hell, the os vulvae, and earth.*

De Graaf was in his twenties when he published *On the organs of women which serve the purpose of procreation* (1672, but not translated from Latin into English until three hundred years later) and, like the rest of the medical profession, worried about possible accusations of salacious activity and so was at pains to say that he 'described the genital parts, not to encourage seduction, and indulgence in pleasure but to improve men's knowledge of themselves for the benefit of the medical community'. His work was more detailed and revelatory than any work previously published on sex and his ideas were laid out meticulously with beautiful, credible anatomical drawings. He was the first to elaborate on the clitoris in detail: whereas, previously, it had been understood as a small penis, a nugatory quasi-male appendage, he emphasized its difference and abundant innervation and function. 'The glans of the clitoris', he wrote, 'is endowed with such sharpened perceptive sensitivity that it is not without justice called the sweetness of love, the gad-fly of Venus'. If it hadn't such an exquisite sensitivity then he imagined that 'no woman would be willing to take upon herself the irksome nine-months-long business of gestation, the painful and often fatal process of expelling the fetus and the worrisome and care-ridden task of raising children'. So women were necessarily lubriciously libidinous, experiencing as much pleasure as men for a good reason, especially 'those females who, with lascivious thoughts, frisky fingers or instruments devised contrary to decent morals, wickedly stir themselves up to such a pitch' that they ejaculate as men do. De Graaf was possibly the first to discover the G-spot (not described until two hundred years later by Gräfenberg) and thought the vagina was so cleverly constructed that it could suit 'each and every penis; it will grow out to meet a short one, retire before a long one, dilate for a fat one, and constrict for a thin one'. Women, fascinating as they might be, were designed for the convenience of men (he also described 'albumen in women's eggs' which could be 'quite prettily demonstrated by boiling them', using the same methods as many of his peers to make his discoveries, that is, an empirical, hands-on experiment, which in this case meant cooking and eating the eggs from a cadaver).

The clitoris has been the object of interest to some and scorn to others over the years: In the 1650s, Nicholas Culpeper, English botanist, herbalist, physician and astrologer, thought it was just like a penis in that it could be erect and a source of 'unspeakable Delight'; yet in the 1980s a medical historian called it 'a minor appendage of the genitalia'. Pinning it down has been controversial, too: in America in 1629, one Thomas or Thomasine Hall was intimately inspected by various worthies – 'I will see what thou carriest' – to determine his/her sex once and for all. She/he dressed as a woman, was 'reported to bee a woman' but was 'proved to bee a man'. Hermaphrodites were considered criminal, or the offspring of crime, since they went against ideas of 'natural' sex, both in law and general understanding. Hall had had sex with 'Greate Besse' and, if proved to be a man, would be guilty of fornication, but if proved a woman, would be guilty of an 'unnatural act'. In effect he/she would be criminalized just by virtue of his/her body, whatever the result of the inspections.

The physician Nicolas de Venette's *The Mysteries of Conjugal Love Reveal'd* (1687) attempted to balance unruly sexuality with religious imperatives, treading a fine line between defusing anxieties and keeping desire within the law. To avoid accusations of obscenity he suggested an offended reader 'should rather accuse his own Lewdness than the words'. The book was Europe's most popular sex manual for the next two hundred years, running to thirty-one editions in France by 1800, and translated into English, German, Dutch and Spanish. Scientific and bawdy, it unveiled everything from African erotic habits to autopsy reports, from Christian pieties to how to recognize an absent maidenhead. It also addressed the age-old question of which sex has the most pleasure, suggesting that women have less but it might last longer for: she is 'the more moist', has a lascivious imagination and a 'great Bum and fleshy thighs'. Medical treatises of this period regularly asked the same question: Martin Schurig in *Spermatologia Historica-Medica* (1720) and *Gynaecologia Historica-Medica* (1730) sat on the fence with 'Many doubts remain', as did W. A. Hammond a hundred years later, believing the question unanswerable, 'and it will remain so as long as we are unable to be men and women alternately'.

Female Sexuality

Anxiety over female sexuality can be found in ancient tradition of literature and art: tales of vagina dentate, one with teeth, and vagina loquens, one that speaks, are significant and symbolic themes. The tales involve obvious fears of castration or being consumed, and talking vaginas may admit to or inform on indiscretions and lovers. They appear early on in French literature: in the thirteenth-century comic verse, *Le Chevalier qui faisoit parler les cons et les culs* (The Knight who made cunts and assholes speak); and in Diderot's 1748 novel *Les Bijoux Indiscrets*, (The Indiscreet Jewels), an allegory portraying Louis XV as the Sultan of the Congo with a magic ring that can make vaginas speak. They chatter on in the American Ozark folk story, *The Magic Walking Stick*, appear in the French film *Le Sexe Qui Parle* (1975) and feature in the contemporary show, The Vagina Monologues.

The infamous, anonymous, and extraordinarily popular *Aristotle's Masterpiece* appeared in 1684 but, unlike Venette, its author had no pretensions to medical research. It enthusiastically records sexual anecdotes, perversities, and a linguistically sensual description of 'secret parts': a woman's 'Seat of Lust [that] excellent Piece of Nature that we are to lay open [is] fresh and red ... like Myrtle Berries'. The 'Clytoris is essential to a woman's pleasure' which 'by swelling up causes Titillation and Delight in those Parts' and is like 'the Comb of a Cock [and] grows sometimes out of the Body two Inches, but that happens not but upon some extraordinary Accident'. It is almost equal in lust to the male 'yard' and, as to the testicles, 'their Number and Place is obvious (there are two of 'em) like a Bunch of Grapes'. The book was still an aid to arousal in the nineteenth century: the Rev. Edward Drax Free of Sandy, Bedfordshire, was defrocked by the church courts for showing his copy of *Aristotle's Masterpiece* to the serving girls he picked up in London, brought home to his rural parish, seduced and impregnated.

The Language of Sex

Distinct terminology began to appear with the 'Rise of Science' in the late-eighteenth century, but it has always been challenged by popular and slang terms, which offer humour and feeling as well as description, and ordinary language arguably gives greater clarification. Antonio Vignali, a sixteenth-century writer, was already poking fun at polite squeamishness in La Cazzaria (The Book of the Prick): 'So when I say priapum, mentual, nervum, you, the reader, will prefer not to believe that these actually mean "cock". Similarly, when you read the words cunnum and vulvum, you will prefer not to recognize them as meaning "cunt".'

Alongside the spread of sexual knowledge was the even more startling spread of sexual diseases, especially syphilis. What is understood by syphilis has changed over time and the disease itself has changed, too: its manifestations and the bacteria that causes it have evolved, as have the perceptions surrounding it. Known as 'the queen of the venereal diseases' (until its dethronement by AIDS), syphilis spread fast and wide, arousing fear and vehemence in medical and political writings, and scurrilous gossip and moral approbation amongst the public. The first medical depictions appeared in 1498. The only prophylactics were abstinence and the condom, the only treatment was mercury, leading to the adage: 'A night with Venus, a lifetime with Mercury'. Condoms were originally made from oiled silk paper, linen, leather, very thin hollow horn, and sheep guts – 'fine seamless membranes of skin' – already in common use as a remedy against a 'big belly' and a 'squawling brat', and now against syphilis, too.

The marks of syphilis, 'purple flowers', were evident on the faces of the afflicted, even on apparently celibate priests and also a pope. Tertiary syphilis (the late phase which may appear years after the first infection) develops in about a third of untreated cases, destroying skin, mucous membranes, internal organs and bones, including nasal and palate bones, leading to terrible disfigurements and to the 'softening of the brain'. The sixteenth-century physician to Pope Alexander VI, Gaspar Torella, advised that if a penis was ulcerated it should be washed thoroughly with soft soap or applied to a cock or a pigeon previously plucked and flayed alive, or perhaps a live frog cut in two. Women were usually regarded as the main contaminators by virtue of their low status and because they were seen as inherently pathological and unclean: physicians sometimes linked infection to 'corrupt' menstrual blood. Different peoples blamed the disease on each other and had different names for it: the Japanese and East Indies knew it as the Portuguese sickness, the French as the English disease, and the English as the French pox. It spread with wars and trade, accompanying troop movements, disrupted populations and behaviours, and its incidence eventually peaked during the early to mid-twentieth century, between the World Wars. Sex and death – Eros and Thanatos – are ancient bedfellows, along with excitement, furtive shame and prejudice. 'Fear of the pox is the beginning of wisdom', wrote one doctor, equating ignorance with promiscuity. By 1944, penicillin was the

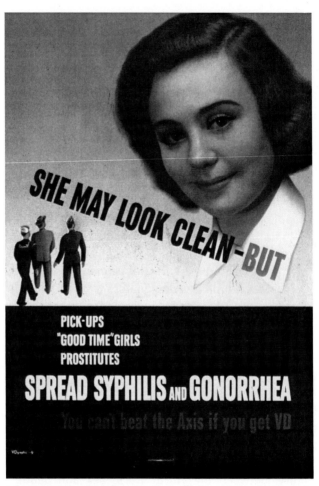

▲ A propaganda poster from the Social Welfare History Archives of the University of Minnesota.
Image Courtesy of The Advertising Archives.

drug of choice for American and British soldiers. It was successful in 90–97 per cent of cases and undoubtedly helped the war effort. Antibiotics have now virtually eradicated tertiary syphilis.

A list of prominent syphilitics includes John Wilmot, Casanova, Beethoven, Schubert, James Boswell (who underwent nineteen bouts of the pox over thirty years), Baudelaire, Gustave Flaubert (who, in 1850, wrote to a friend saying that in Cairo 'One admits one's sodomy, and it is spoken of at table in the hotel ... we have considered it our duty to indulge in this form of ejaculation'), Guy de Maupassant, Oscar Wilde, James Joyce, Nietzsche, Van Gogh, Paul Gauguin, and Randolph Churchill, who gave his last speech in 1894 before suffering 'a general paralysis of the insane'. Women, of course, caught syphilis too, though you might not think it from the usual lists; they lacked the bravado that many men seemed to accord themselves when infected and risked losing more than their minds before the disease killed them. They didn't proclaim their infamy, unlike Guy de Maupassant who died in an asylum in 1893 aged forty-two:

I've got the pox!

He proclaimed this proudly in a letter, continuing, 'At last! Not the contemptible clap ... the majestic pox ... and I'm proud of it ... I don't have to worry about catching it anymore, and I screw the street whores and trollops, and afterwards I say to them, "I've got the pox". They are afraid and I just laugh'.

This hostility towards the prostitutes he frequented was perhaps a revenge for his infection, for the blame game where sexual diseases are concerned is nothing new. When Josephine Butler fought the 'social purity' campaign against the Contagious Diseases Act in the 1860s, she was attacking an unjust legislation that punished women, the 'victims of vice and [left] unpunished the sex who are the main cause'.

English church courts were attempting to cement social and sexual stratification in the seventeenth century, with up to 90 per cent of the cases brought concerning fornication, adultery, sodomy and prostitution, and the punishments meted out could be savage. The sexual behaviour of the general population was proving hard to control and the sensational sexual scandals of the aristocracy even more so. The most extraordinary case involved Mervyn Touchet, 2nd Earl of Castlehaven, beheaded in 1631 for committing 'almost every known sexual felony'. At his trial it was claimed that he had arranged, among other things, for his wife to be raped by a servant and that he had committed sodomy with a manservant, Florence (or Lawrence) Fitzpatrick. Castlehaven's case was brought as codes of sexual morality were tightening and Puritans were gaining ideological ground. The 'spiritual authority' of Puritanism, challenged by the Restoration that followed the Civil War of the 1640s, tends now to signify repression, though in the 1600s it was a reform movement of dissenters who wanted to simplify and purify the Church, do away with Catholic idolatry and emphasize a personal interpretation of the Bible. It was also responsible for a 'masculinization' of sexuality, interpreting women as objects, as 'Other', and forging a sexual ideology that conflated female chastity with female identity. Sexuality was appropriated by men, thus restricting the acceptable roles of women to wife and mother – and though sex outside wedlock was frowned upon, it happened anyway and was made respectable through marriage. Religious and State regulations, moral and economic conditions all had bearing on sexual behaviour but they didn't always hold sway.

Female petitioners to Parliament in the English Civil War were dismissed and insulted as 'Whores, Bawdes, Oyster-women, Irish women' – political pornographia (from the Greek *pornē*: the prostitute, and *graphē*: the recorded mark or sign, verbal or visual). There were plenty of names in use that could demean or ruin a woman simply by referring to her sex and making a mockery of her (just as there are today). Words such as queane, punke, drab, flurt, strumpet, harlot, cockatrice, naughty pack, light housewife, and common hackney were commonplace. Attitudes to actual prostitutes celebrated or denigrated depended on the social sphere she inhabited: she might be a royal mistress, pleasure-seeking wife, or high-class courtesan, such as the character Angellica Bianca in Aphra Behn's play, *The Rover* (1677), displaying her status and advertising her enormous fees. *The Rover* showed the sexual and social constraints women faced where, according to one critic, 'ladies act like whores and whores like ladies', though this comment merely revealed the two principal definitions of women: virgin and whore. There was no room for the sexually free, independent female. Women often wore masks to Restoration plays, either because the plays were so crude that they couldn't watch them in mixed company with their faces uncovered or, possibly, to pick up men. Some suggested that it was a perverse desire of 'modish women' to be seen as whores [viz. today, Miley Cyrus, etc.]. The Restoration Libertines, even if they allowed for a ribald female sexuality, could not be said to have been free of double standards: Claude Le Petit, a libertine executed at the stake in 1662 aged just twenty-three, had written a graphic sonnet to the '"Cortisanes d'honneur" inviting them to use his manuscript as a dildo.'

John Wilmot, Earl of Rochester – *The Imperfect Enjoyment*

This dart of love, whose piercing point, oft tried...

Which nature still directed with such art

That it through every cunt reached every heart—

Stiffly resolved, 'twould carelessly invade

Woman or man, nor aught its fury stayed:

Where'er it pierced, a cunt it found or made

In the mid-eighteenth century, a backlash against Puritanism in much of Europe amounted to a sexual revolution. With the Restoration had come a swing of the pendulum, from licence to repression and back to licence again, and it allowed works such those by the libertine poet John Wilmot, the Earl of Rochester.

Rochester, the witty, rakish son of a Cavalier hero, was a favourite of Charles II, despite accusing the king of being obsessed with sex and neglecting his country. Rochester was writing his bawdy verse as the sexually explicit Restoration comedies hit the theatres and *Aristotle's Masterpiece* was published (despite the 1662 Licensing Act in England for suppression of indecent publications – there was a vagueness about the definition of 'indecent', as there is of 'obscene' today). Puritanism had begun to lose its fierce grip, at least on the nation's imagination.

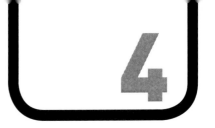

Savagery and tenderness

For spirits when they please

*Can either sex assume,
or both; so soft*

*And uncompounded is their
essence pure*

John Milton

The eighteenth-century Enlightenment had a major influence on our modern culture of sex. New ideas and models led to policy-making, and individual sexuality acquired a new level of distinctiveness. A process of cementing them now began. A plethora of medical essays, anatomical illustrations, midwifery books and religio-political texts describing and commenting on sexuality and sexual behaviour were published. Daniel Defoe's essay 'Conjugal Lewdness or, Matrimonial Whoredom' (1727) was, despite its title, a rant against contraception: the whoredom came from the enjoyment of sex for the sake of it (the term 'contraception' wouldn't appear until 1919, in Max Marcuse's *The Sexual Meaning of Procreation and Contraception* (1919); he suggested other terms, too, including 'spermathanaton' – sperm death). Parson Thomas Malthus published *An Essay on the Principle of Population* (1798) arguing that human misery was a consequence of rapid population growth, though contemporary works such as *The Secrets of the Alcove* were available, detailing contraceptive methods for popular use. Contemporary methods included keeping your eyes shut or drinking milk during sex, and trying different positions, such as the woman on top.

Novels portraying ribald sexuality were widely read too: the infamous English erotic novel, *Fanny Hill: or, the Memoirs of a Woman of Pleasure* (1749), was translated into many European languages (there were fourteen French editions by the end of the eighteenth century) and it had many imitators. Written by John Cleland while he was incarcerated in Fleet prison for his debts, it was an enormous success, allowing him to pay back what he owed, but then reducing him again to penury because of its perceived obscenity.

Sexually explicit works are an intrinsic part of Western culture and have emphasized and perpetuated fundamental categories and ideas about different sexualities. *Fanny Hill* is a man's idea of female sexuality. Some have suggested that Cleland was homosexual – he was supposed to be a sodomite, and his erstwhile friend, Thomas Cannon ('that execrable, white-faced, rotten catamite', according to Cleland), had published an early defence of homosexuality, *Ancient and Modern Pederasty Investigated and Exemplify'd* (1749) – for which the publisher was imprisoned as Cannon fled the country.

In Cleland's novel, Fanny comes across two sodomites having sex and tells her bawd, Mrs Cole, who says they are:

stript of all the manly virtues of their own sex and fill'd up with only the very worst vices and follies of ours; that in fine, they were scarce less execrable than ridiculous in their monstrous inconsistency, of loathing and condemning women, and all at the same time, apeing their manners, airs, lisp, skuttle.

Then, as now, despite its ubiquity in homosexual and heterosexual relations, there was a great deal of fearful hostility towards sodomy and sodomites. It was a prejudice exacerbated by canonical law, civil law, and theology, all of which centred on the prescribed union of marriage – not that sex within marriage wasn't rule-bound, too.

Many thought of sodomy as a conveniently 'foreign practice'; in 1727 an English clergyman wrote that it 'rarely appears in our Histories' and then only 'among Monsters and Prodigies'. In early eighteenth-century London, however, 'molly houses' were common and men might be 'completely rigged in gowns, petticoats, headcloths, fine laced shoes, furbelowed scarves, and masks; some had riding hoods, some were dressed like milkmaids and others like shepherdesses with green hats ... and others had their faces patched and painted and wore very extensive hoop petticoats'. Cannon had argued that 'Unnatural Desire is a Contradiction in Terms; downright Nonsense', but to be a sodomite was to have an essential identity, such as race and gender. This setting apart of a specific, 'unnatural' dimension of sexuality can be interpreted, according to Foucault, as a leaning towards more liberal ideas or towards a more strict supervision of behaviour.

Contemporary discussion among an educated elite claiming the authority of knowledge also functioned as ideology as a way of describing the 'norm', such as what is expected of whom, what is or is not sanctioned, or the distinctions made between men and women. That is not to say a prevailing idea couldn't be subverted by the different behaviours and observations of the general population, or those who had alternative knowledge and beliefs about sexuality. Diderot, encyclopaedist, atheist, philosopher and libertine, believed that no sexual behaviour, from incest to bestiality, was inherently immoral or unnatural. His posthumously published dialogues (1760s) attacked European sexual mores, comparing them to Polynesian sexual attitudes and practices: these were nature's children perplexed by imported French inhibitions. While Diderot was arguing that 'There is a bit of testicle at the bottom of our most sublime feeling and our purest tenderness', men were being executed for sodomy in England. Execution for this act continued until 1835: forty-six were executed between 1810 and 1835 and a further thirty-two were condemned but reprieved, while over seven hundred got off with a milder sentence. In France, the last execution for sodomy was in 1783, not long after Thomas Jefferson had recommended that sodomitic women in America had holes cut in their noses (only in 2003 did the US Supreme Court strike down all Texan sodomy laws). Jefferson was just as dogmatic towards the sexual behaviour of Native American men: when it became known that indigenous Americans rarely raped their female captives (a common practice amongst Europeans) it was said that they had 'no ardour [and] little sexual capacity'. Jefferson thought otherwise; that their sexuality was savage, that they had no capacity for 'tender delicate' feeling, and so were 'abnormal' and not, as in the 'normal' Christian ideal, heterosexual and monogamous.

Women who loved other women were largely ignored, though they were discreet. Some lived together as a married couple, some lived dressed as men, others became soldiers and sailors and their sex was only discovered when they died or were punished by the lash. The twice-married Mary Delaney (1700–1788), friend of Hogarth, Swift and Handel, had many intimate women friends – sometimes sexual and sometimes chaste – in London and Dublin. After the death of her second husband, she spent her time with the Duchess of Portland designing an erotic garden for her.

Delaney's contemporary, Dr Samuel Johnson (1709–1783), tried to persuade his biographer, the diarist James Boswell, that 'keeping a mistress as well as a wife' went against the 'duties of morality and religion and the dignity of human nature'. It brought 'confusion and misery into society; and it is a transgression of the laws of the Almighty Creator, who has ordained marriage for the mutual comfort of the sexes and the procreation and right educating of children'. Boswell tried, but failed, to conform. There were, after all, a 'variety of fine girls' along the Strand 'all wearing Venus's girdle' offering 'amorous intercourse'. He vowed not to return to London without his wife, but later caved in and told her that he 'must have a concubine. She said I might go to whom I pleased. She has often said so'. Boswell's diary is full of his exploits, one of which illustrates the closeness of sex and death: in 1784 he attended the execution of nineteen felons, and went on to Betsy Smith's to tell her '"I have got a shocking sight in my head, take it out" ... Her pleasing vivacity *did* remove it'.

Japanese Erotic Art

During the Edo period, C17–C19, Japan was quite isolated and had developed a different sexual and moral landscape – sex was not aligned with sin, cruelty or violence, and there was little in the way of objectification, even though the position of women was lowly. Japanese shunga ('spring pictures') erotic paintings, prints and books by artists of the ukiyo-e ('floating world' school) turned authority and hierarchy upside down and celebrated sexuality in explicitly fine and colourful detail, emphasizing humour and sensuality. The artists were mainly male artists but their work was enjoyed by men and women of all classes, though they were banned in Japan for much of the twentieth century. Artists such as Utamaro, Hokusai and Kunisada inspired European artists, including Toulouse-Lautrec, Beardsley, Rodin and Picasso. Shunga continues to inspire Japanese art, from tattoo work to manga and anime. The ars erotica of societies such as China, Japan, India, Rome, and Arabo-Moslem have been compared and likened to Western scientia sexualis.

In the 1790s, as the French Revolution caused tremors of fear across Europe, the Marquis de Sade's (1740–1814) erotic writings were combining philosophy and sexual violence, fantasy, freedom and blasphemy – much of it written in prison or the insane asylum. De Sade was eventually turned in by prostitutes outraged by his unconventional use of a communion wafer. In Italy, Casanova (1725–1798) also languished in prison for outrages against the Church, and while there he wrote a detailed and revealing autobiography, *Histoire de ma vie jusqu'à l'an*, revealing some of the sexual customs

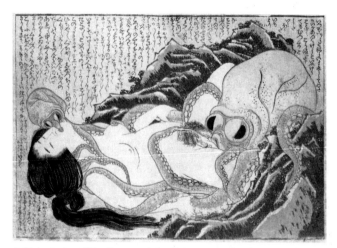

▲ 'Tako to Ama (The Dream of the Fisherman's Wife)' Hokusai, 1814

and established mores of life in eighteenth-century Europe – though it was not published in full until 1960. His name has become a byword for philandering men and, though he appreciated intelligent women for their 'simple reasoning [and] delicacy of feeling', he thought them incapable of true learning as it would 'compromise the essential qualities of her sex'. Promiscuous and unscrupulous, he did always use 'assurance caps' or the 'fines redingotes d'Angleterre' (English raincoat) to prevent disease and pregnancies while he 'overwhelmed them with happiness for several hours'.

Ideas on childhood sexuality also began to come under scrutiny in the eighteenth century – ideas which have changed through societies and time, often through the need to establish boundaries for such steps as marriage, consent, and giving evidence in court.

Childhood sexuality as a separate sphere was not much regarded before 1700; physicians in general ignored it, apart from writing about masturbation, the form of sexuality most associated with children. Ideas about which bodies could appropriately engage in sex were informed by age, physical constitution and formation, or gender, and were dictated by physical maturity and whether reproduction was possible. Children, pre-puberty, were considered 'unripe', and it followed that they must be unacquainted with sexual feeling, desire and pleasure. It was thought, however, that they could be acquainted, sexualized through contact, ointments and 'remedies', but that this was a deviation and was treated as such in prosecutions for rape or fornication. In *The Secret Miracle of Nature* (1658), Levinus Lemnius wrote that at puberty there 'ariseth a ticklish delight, and itching in their inward parts, and they begin to burn in love, and are easily allured to copulation'. Jane Sharp, in her *Midwives Book* (1671), stated that 'generally maids have their terms at fourteen years old [their] breasts swell; lustful thoughts draw away their minds, and some fall into Consumptions, others rage and grow almost mad with love'. Boys reached puberty at a similar age or slightly later, 'they have much vitall strength, and their secrets begin to be hairy, and their chins begin to shoot forth, with fine decent down, which force and heat of procreating Children increaseth daily' (i.e. their ability to ejaculate). Sexuality, it was believed, appeared with physical maturity.

The age of consent has been central to ideas about the nature of childhood, and first appeared – set at twelve years, the legal age of marriage – in secular law in 1275 in England as part of the rape law, though judgements were often made on the appearance and behaviour of girls and whether they seemed sufficiently child-like or a victim. The late eighteenth-century Enlightenment concept of childhood, based on physical development, led to other European nations enacting age of consent laws: the Napoleonic code established an age of consent of eleven in 1791, which applied to boys as well as girls. This was raised to thirteen in France in 1863, and 1865 in England. Twenty years later, W. T. Stead's series of articles in the *Pall Mall Gazette*, 'The Maiden Tribute of Modern Babylon', a controversial exposé of child prostitution, caused a sensational outcry, and the subsequent raising of the age of consent to sixteen. Boys and youths were generally thought of as sexual agents and not victims. In America, arguments over the law dwelt on new scientific data on whether psychological maturity came later than physiological maturity, and whether girls could enter into contracts and hold property rights, but it was all muddied by accusations that teenage girls were sufficiently developed not to need legal protection and might use the law to blackmail unwary men. In India, the British applied the age of consent to married as well as unmarried girls – child marriage was traditional among Hindus – and created a crime of marital rape that did not exist in British law. The 1860 Indian Penal Code set the age at ten years, reflecting ideas that non-white races 'matured earlier', effectively 'ripening' more quickly in hot climates. In America, there were similar ideas about African-Americans, Mexicans, and Italian immigrants.

The world-wide average age of consent is 16, though there are dramatic international differences: the appropriate age for sex in Yemen is as young as 9, as long as there are signs of the 'onset of puberty'; while in Tunisia, unmarried couples must be 20 years old. In Austria, Italy and Germany, the age of consent is 14; in Sweden, France and Denmark it is 15, and it is 16 in Spain, where the age of consent was recently raised from 13. In Turkey and Malta, young people must wait until they are 18 for sex to be legal. The law in Canada is more nuanced; they raised the age of consent from 14 to 16, but the law criminalizes older 'predators' while not prosecuting younger teenagers in similar age relationships. This means that children of 12 can legally have sex as long as neither partner is more than two years older than the other, and the age of consent rises to 18 if one partner is in a position of power. In Britain, the age of consent for homosexual males was lowered to 18 in 1979, and in 2000 was lowered to 16, the same as for heterosexuals. The third National Survey of Sexual Attitudes and Lifestyles (Natsal), published in 2013, has the UK median average age of first sexual experience also as 16; it has remained the same since the 2000 survey, and the number of people having sex before that age has not differed significantly either (31 per cent of men and 29 per cent of women). Some countries make a point of differentiating between heterosexuals and homosexuals, but for the age of consent for heterosexual relationships most countries have focused on the behaviour of girls.

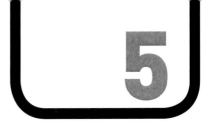

Sexuality meets Science

It sounds like a scientific fairy-tale

Richard Krafft-Ebing

Speculation about sexuality was rife in the nineteenth century, and ideas and arguments about race, the origin of the family, morality, religion, law and private property were endlessly developed and debated. This was a time of pathologizing and categorizing sexual behaviours and preferences, most of which were seen as aberrant and often a sign of insanity – for example, homosexuality, masturbation, and fetishes. There were differences between 'high' and 'low' sexual knowledge, and tense connections between popular and scientific ideas. Experience, experimentation, danger, vulgarity and sheer variety vied with regulation, description and an avalanche of respectability. Moral panics, such as the 'anti-speculum crusade', took off. Pioneering figures such as Josephine Butler campaigned against sexual double standards and the Contagious Diseases Act between 1869 and 1886. The term 'pornography', defined as we understand it today, appeared in the Oxford English Dictionary in 1857. A sea-change in knowledge and sensibilities arrived – the ancient idea that women needed to orgasm in order to conceive began to lose general favour (though in 2012, Republican Senator Todd Akin revealed that he still believed in it), and a greater social stratification of delights led to cross-overs between upper and lower classes, which was a taboo in itself.

Sexuality was becoming a serious subject for serious men unafraid of its 'loathsome aspects'. People were increasingly defined by their sexuality as it became harder to extricate the quasi-science from the sex manual: in the 1860s the eminent surgeon and moralist William Acton, for example, replaced inquisitive desire with erotic insanity, especially in women, stating that 'The majority (happily for society) are not very much troubled with sexual feelings of any kind'. The emerging sexology attempted to prevail with order and categories, but was undermined by its hysterical approach to the female body, its moral manacles, and its psychiatrization of all pleasures apparently perverse. Teachers, parents, police, politicians and priests were called upon to educate the thousands of 'thoughtless, passionate, habitually licentious men' and Paphian women who, under a 'veil of that artificial bashfulness', were allegedly indulging themselves in lubricious erotomania. But all was not lost, as long as popular appetite remained unsated there were those who did not 'object to dealing with filth' in order to dispel ignorance and prejudice, almost a 'pornography of the morbid'. There was a drive for 'truth', albeit a Western truth, about sexuality, a *scientia sexualis*.

Sexuality was not a fount of sin and transgression alone; it was also said to make you ill, and doctors were discovering and treating all manner of physical and psychological sicknesses that resulted from thinking about, let alone having, unconventional sex. 'Normal' adult, heterosexual reproductive sex was the ideal, and the authorities sought to promote it. According to Foucault, at the beginning of the eighteenth century there were four determining strategic sources of sexual knowledge and power:

1 The hysterization of women's bodies: the feminine body was analysed and pathologized – qualified and disqualified – as though saturated with sexuality.

2 The pedagogization of children's sex: the assertion that most children indulge in or are prone to sexual activity, especially masturbation, was deemed contrary to 'nature' and rife with physical and moral dangers, both for them and for society.

3 The socialization of procreative behaviour: the economic socialization of incitement and restrictions brought to bear on fertility of couples.

4 The psychiatrization of perverse pleasure: the sex instinct was isolated as a separate biological and psychical instinct; clinically analysed and assigned as normal, aberrant or pathological behaviour which required correction.

Darwin's *The Origin of Species* (1859) was a sudden jolt to society as the argument that human sexuality was an animalistic behaviour made 'civilized' sex begin to look like a thin veneer. It was greeted with distaste and disgust. People also regarded it with humour and relief, but mostly with disgust. Academic argument was busy setting out criteria of sexuality, and their results reflected their preconceptions about themselves and about non-Western people whom they assumed were over-sexed because they were more 'primitive'. Evolutionary social theory had it that there existed a base line of sexual promiscuity, where not even incest was taboo, from which peoples progressed at different rates towards the European ideal of monogamous, bourgeois marriage. Friedrich Engels (1820–1895), a German social scientist, argued that primitive sexual free-for-all could not support a system of private property, and only by restricting women within the family was this made possible. Engels wanted a better future, and his theories were used to explore the ideal of free love in the Soviet Union. Free-love movements which shun marriage as a form of slavery have come and gone over the centuries. Russian experimental communities were wound up in the 1920s when Stalin took over the Communist Party, bringing in more conservative policies. In Japan, members of a free-love movement were executed in the Amakasu Incident in 1923. In England, thinkers such as William Blake, Mary Wollstonecraft and Bertrand Russell were high-profile exponents of free love, and Victoria Woodhull (1838–1927), 'the high priestess of free love', was the first woman to run for presidency in the US. She wrote:

'Yes, I am a Free Lover. I have an inalienable, constitutional and natural right to love whom I may, to love as long or as short a period as I can; to change that love every day if I please, and with that right neither you nor any law you can frame have any right to interfere. And I have the further right to demand a free and unrestricted exercise of that right, and it is your duty not only to accord it, but, as a community, to see that I am protected in it. I trust that I am fully understood, for I mean just that, and nothing less!'.

The Oneida Perfectionists

The Oneida Perfectionists were a Utopian community led by John Humphrey Noyes in the mid-nineteenth century, one of many communities in the Puritan utopian model established two hundred years before. Noyes experienced a religious conversion during the Second Great Awakening (the first was Calvinist) when thousands of Americans were reacting to great social and political changes. The Awakening looked back to what seemed a simple, golden age and Noyes preached inner salvation and the realization of the Kingdom of Heaven on earth: his community would duplicate Heaven, all would be equal and there would be 'complex marriage'. The idea was to instil love and loyalty through free love and multiple partners for all men and women. They practised 'male continence' or *coitus reservatus*, a form of birth control as well as social engineering – stirpiculture – a proto-eugenic experiment in breeding good stock that meant that only the 'best' would parent children. Noyes founded his first controversial community in Putney, Vermont, in 1840, but they were forced out pending arrests for adultery. They moved to Oneida, NY, in 1848, but the community failed and many members returned to conventional marriage and child-rearing. Utopian communities also had strong ties with feminism and spiritualism.

Control of sexuality seemed vital to social order and evolutionary advance, and seemed evident when the British looked to the different behaviours of their colonial subjects: there was an invention of the 'primitive' and a newly emerging concept of 'race' in which 'savages' appeared to live in a state of sexual immorality that justified their subjugation. Lust was 'the heart of darkness', and colonial officials and missionaries regarded the habit of nakedness as lustful, whereas the naked thought the authorities ludicrous for wearing their woollen suits in tropical heat. Anthropologists understood the sexuality of those they studied according to their Euro-American understandings, and allotted titles to these behaviours: perversion, inversion, homosexuality, adultery, norm, marriage, transvestism. This was often quite baffling to the people being characterized, analysed, and 'normalized', by their colonial masters who used sexuality as a stick with which to beat the local populations. In Western Australia, wrote the anthropologist R. H. Matthews, a circumcised man would be 'given' the uncircumcised brother of the woman he would later marry and 'used [him] for purposes of masturbation and sodomy'. Reports of 'primitive' open sexuality, polygamy, and circumcision in the colonies fed back into social science and were absorbed by the press, leading to anxiety-drenched stories about the underclass of London's East End where similar degeneracy also apparently existed – as recorded by Henry Mayhew in *London Labour and the London Poor* (1861–2) which contained tales of thieves, beggars, prostitutes, and premarital and extramarital sex. However, it was mostly an anecdotal, second-hand account.

In the eighteenth century, when savage tribes in various parts of the world first began to be visited, extravagantly romantic views widely prevailed as to the simple and idyllic lives led by primitive peoples. During the greater part of the nineteenth century, the tendency of opinion was to the opposite extreme, and it became usual to insist on the degraded and licentious morals of savages ... In reality, however, savage life is just as little a prolonged debauch as a protracted idyll.

Havelock Ellis, a British physician and social reformer, Studies in the Psychology of Sex, *1897–1928.*

The Hottentot Venus

Saartjie Baartman was made famous in Europe as The Hottentot Venus (1789–1815). She had been brought from South Africa to London in 1810 and became the object of salacious exploitation and scientific interest for Europeans. As a young girl she had been widowed and orphaned on the same day, later becoming a servant to a showman, Hendrik Cesars, who then took her to London hoping to make money from her in a semi-naked display upon the stage. The British were fascinated by her huge buttocks and her genitalia, fabled to be equally disproportionate, at a time when political satire was taken up with all things posterior. Although campaigners sought to free Saartjie from the circus that surrounded her, Cesars had made a deal with a French showman in 1815 and Saartjie was soon taken up by the celebrated naturalist Georges Cuvier, becoming the object of his sexual and scientific interest. She died in the December of that year and he dissected her body in what her biographer calls a 'hypersexual post-mortem'.

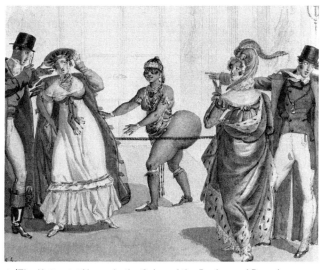

▲ 'The Hottentot Venus in the Salon of the Duchess of Berry', Sebastien Coeure, 1830
The Hottentot Venus in the Salon of the Duchess of Berry, 1830 (w/c on paper), Coeure, Sebastien (1778–p.1831) / Private Collection / Archives Charmet / The Bridgeman Art Library

Richard Krafft-Ebing's *Psychopathia Sexualis* (1886) categorized behaviours and desires from adultery to lesbianism to zooerasty, distinguishing between the 'healthy' and the 'degenerate' as though applying some order might put the sexes 'back in their proper places'. This approach was an early form of psychobiology, the interconnection of mental and physiological functions; in Krafft-Ebbing's scheme, sadism and masochism, for example, were inherent – sadism being the extreme form of the male tendency to dominate, and masochism was at the other end of spectrum with the female desire to submit – and where unacknowledged sexual currents of Christian asceticism ran deep. Even though sexology was shaped by Christian culture and the idea of agony and ecstasy was culturally ingrained, mortification of the flesh, for example, was now reinterpreted as a self-deceiving way of achieving sexual gratification. Categorization and regulation, always changing, always with us, was now backed by the authority of science. Havelock Ellis, an essentialist, saw human sexuality as a biological given, as opposed to the constructionist view that prevails today where shared meanings and choices create traditions of thought and behaviour. He advocated better treatment for those whose sexuality did not fit the norm, believing homosexuality to be natural, and that male and female same-sex relations should be legalized. His own sexuality was unconventional: his wife Edith was openly lesbian, their union unconsummated, and he was aroused by urolagnia (watching women pee). Havelock Ellis was brave to publish and speak out: in 1897, when his work *Sexual Inversion* came out (based on letters he had received and on the writings of the poet John Addington Symonds), its publisher was sent to prison and the remaining volumes had to be taken over by an American medical publisher.

There is no shortage of examples showing 'other', or deviant, behaviours in the Victorian period, but there were few without censure at a time when sexual desire itself was considered debilitating. Questions of medico-legal intervention were aligned with perversions, criminality, and theories of inherited degeneration: was the perceived problem one of contagion and corruption or was it an innate predisposition? 'Paraphilia' was a new early twentieth-century term to describe 'perversion', perhaps a less judgemental word but still linked to ideas of degeneration (from the classical notion of the loss of vital spirits through ejaculation), and the moral, physiological and mental decay of individual and nation. Paraphilias are conditions in which sexual arousal and gratification depends on fantasizing about or acting on behaviours or objects that are atypical, and sometimes viewed as extreme. Different behaviours are described as paraphiliac at different times and may be centred on an object of erotic interest (a shoe, fabrics, or a car) or a particular act that arouses (vomiting or watching someone crying), but they are mainly desires that societies find unpleasant or unusual. Many are or have been regulated by the law and by moral and religious constraints. Paraphilias are not merely acts, sacred or profane, they are practices that define people as particular types, and where desire and identity may merge. The *Diagnostic and Statistical Manual of Mental Disorders* (DSM) of the American Psychological Association says that when a paraphiliac desire or behaviour causes distress it reveals mental disorder – 'deviance' in itself is not enough. Fetishism (the word derives from the French fétiche, which comes from the Portuguese feitiço, 'spell') is another term denoting sexual arousal from a physical object, and is obsession related to association or substitution (today there are plenty of fetish clubs, fetish fashions, and websites). There is potentially a limitless list of paraphilias, from abasiophilia (a term coined in 1990 to describe psychosexual attraction to those with impaired mobility, perhaps using leg braces, orthopaedic casts or wheelchairs), to nasophilia (sexual fixation on noses; Freud thought the nose was a substitute for the penis), to zoophilia (term introduced by Krafft-Ebing in 1886 to denote sexual attraction to animals). Some paraphilias are harmless but others are potentially dangerous, such as hybristophilia which means sexual arousal dependent upon a partner having committed a violent crime, or asphyxiophilia, the erotic interest in asphyxiation. Nymphomania appeared in the medical dictionary in 1861: 'women who suffer from it give in to licentious acts, lubricious manipulations, and speak in obscene language, announcing their violent arousal and displaying perversions of the instincts génésiques'. Necrophiliacs were diagnosed with vampirism, a term coined in 1850 by Joseph Guislain, a Belgian alienist (psychologist) and clinical reformer: 'It is within the category of the destructive madmen ... not innately different to other "perverts" [just] ... going that bit further than them: "one has to align [the] sad disorders of the reproductive instinct [onanism, nymphomania, satyriasis] with the depraved tastes that prompt certain individuals to profane female and even male cadavers, and to exercise their ghastly passion on them".' George Selwyn, MP (1719–1791) was sexually fascinated with corpses but his peers merely found him odd. When Selwyn called to visit the deathbed of his friend Henry Fox, the dying man reputedly said, 'If Mr. Selwyn calls again, show him up. If I am alive, I shall be glad to see him, and if I am dead, I am sure he will be delighted to see me!'

Dr Isaac Baker Brown believed that excessive desire in women would lead to depravity, derangement and even death, and he became infamous for performing clitoridectomies – surgical excision of the clitoris – in a private London clinic in the 1860s, often without the patient's consent. He would 'set to work to remove [it] whenever he had the opportunity of doing so', according to his obituary in the *Medical Times and Gazette*, and would operate on girls as young as ten years old, as well as women who wanted to take advantage of the 1857 Divorce Act, and women with eye problems. Female circumcision (now known as female genital mutilation, FGM) restricted female sexuality to reproduction alone. As late as 1899 T. C. Allbutt was warning, in *A System of Medicine*, that precocious sexuality would interfere with 'normal' mental growth.

Many of Baker Brown's colleagues saw benefits to his 'occasionally valuable and desirable operation' but he was expelled from the Obstetric Society in 1867 after too many complaints from his patients. The Secretary of the Obstetric Society condemned clitoridectomy as a misuse of male power but believed that the medical profession was there to guard women's interests and honour and, indeed, it could be said to have women at its mercy. He tried to imagine a reversal of the status quo where female doctors argued that 'most of the unmanageable maladies of men were to be traced to some morbid change in their genitals, founding societies for the discussion of them and hospitals for the cure of them, one of them sitting in her consultation chair, with her little stove by her side and her irons all hot, searing every man as he passed before her'.

Male patients who were diagnosed with the alleged condition of satyriasis (overpowering sexual desire in men) very rarely underwent castration. Satyriasis was thought to be a much milder affliction than the corresponding female nymphomania, and where men could be taught to control themselves, women risked a life of prostitution or being confined in an asylum. Female sexuality threatened the fabric of society in a way that male sexuality did not. Male monomanias, inappropriate expressions of masculinity such as the compulsive masturbator, corpse violator or homicidal monomaniac, were worrisome, but male sexual desire was the norm and men were not defined by their reproductive lives or their genitalia.

Hypersexuality

Hypersexuality is said to be extremely frequent sexual urges or activity, or a sudden increase in these, though the condition is not agreed upon and usually the cause is unknown. The World Health Organization's (WHO) International Classification of Diseases lists 'Excessive Sexual Drive' in which 'satyrisis' applies to men and 'nymphomania' to women (it has also been known as Don Juanism, erotomania, and the Messalina complex). The American Psychiatric Association has not so far included hypersexuality in the DSM, its list of psychiatric disorders, and many question whether the alleged condition is a disorder at all, given that labelling some people's urges as 'extreme' merely demonizes those whose sexuality doesn't conform to a norm. Hypersexuality could be due to illnesses such as bipolar or obsessive-compulsive disorders, to dementia, to brain injuries, or to the side-effects of certain medicines and drugs such as alcohol. Hormonal changes may also cause a leap in sexual appetite and behaviour, or even the simplest desire for intimacy. A popular term for hypersexuality is 'sex addiction'.

Krafft-Ebing discussed the potential dangers of sexual desire as a fount of destruction, a force that must be tamed. 'Natural instinct', he believed, was committed to procreation, but he confused class and nature when he wrote, 'if a woman is normally developed mentally and well-bred, her sexual desire is small. If this were not so, the whole world would become a brothel'. Women were pathological if they showed too much interest in sex, of whatever hue. But not everyone agreed. Elizabeth Garrett Anderson accused the male dominated medical profession of misrepresenting female sexuality as diseased and abnormal, and the American journalist and advocate of women's rights, Mary Livermore, called the idea a 'monstrous assumption that woman is a natural invalid' and railed against the 'unclean army of "gynaecologists" who seem desirous to convince women that they possess but one set of organs – and that these are always diseased'. Mary Putnam Jacobi MD wrote in 1895 that *it is in the increased attention paid to women, and especially in their new function as lucrative patients, scarcely imagined a hundred years ago, that we find explanation for much of the ill-health among women, freshly discovered today.*

Even the speculum, an ancient medical instrument (three bronze examples were dug from the ruins of Pompeii in 1818), was said to be a cause of uncontrolled sexual desire in women. In Victorian London an anti-speculum crusade was sparked when it was reported that 'crowds of women rushed to a gentleman's door, begging to have the speculum used'. The instrument was seen as a potential threat to the family as wives and mothers succumbed to this 'new and lamentable form of hysteria' which degraded the pure minds of 'the daughters of England': moodiness and perversion would overcome them, they would stutter incoherently, and might even prefer the doctor and his speculum to a husband's attentions. Speculum use was negatively associated with French syphilitic wards, and while some medics thought that 'a noble nature should aspire after a better world ... where no physician will be required to meddle with delicate organs', others argued that purity was a state of mind that could not be destroyed by physical means. One might conclude that it was the crusade that was hysterical.

Sexuality meets Science

Masturbating in Public

This act remains prohibited in the UK, with up to 14 days in prison, depending on the circumstances. The key law is Section 28 of the Town Police Clauses Act 1847 wherein it is an offence for someone to 'wilfully and indecently' expose his 'person' (i.e. penis) in a street or public place to the obstruction, annoyance or danger of residents or passengers. In Indonesia, the maximum sentence is 32 months imprisonment; in Saudi Arabia, in 2004, a teacher was sentenced to 3 years and 300 lashes for saying that masturbation (and homosexuality, smoking and music) were permissible under Islam; in 2009 in America (where laws vary from state to state) the Supreme Court of Alabama outlawed the sale of 'any device designed ... primarily for the stimulation of human genital organs'.

6

Truth and sexuality

The realization of oneself is the prime aim of life, and to realize oneself through pleasure is finer than to do so through pain ... it is a pagan idea

Oscar Wilde

Not all Victorian sex was so morbidly laden, much pleasure can also be found in private diaries and letters. Take, for example, the mid-nineteenth-century literary and inseparable brothers, Jules and Edmond de Goncourt, who diligently record their lovers' cries as they brought them to orgasm: 'Oh! Bibi, I'm coming ... Hum ... hum ... hum ... Do it! Oh! ... Do it, say, pig! ... Oh! Everything's wet'. 'Hi! hi! hi!' – Snuffly breathing. In low tones: 'That's tickling me nicely ... Push hard ... Ah! Oh! I want to go on top of you ... Oh! My Bibi Oh! you're going too far, my God! ... Your heart was beating under my buttocks'. And, *apropos* George Bernard Shaw, it was marriage that could prove to be the most licentious of human institutions: combining the maximum of temptation with the maximum of opportunity, married couples could, and many did, freely express their sexuality. The young Queen Victoria felt strong sexual and emotional stirrings on first setting eyes on her future consort, Albert: 'He is perfection', she wrote. She thought him excessively handsome with such a pretty mouth, a beautiful figure, broad-shouldered and narrow-waisted; she admired his strength and his weight. On her wedding in 1840, Victoria rapturously told her diary that she had, 'NEVER NEVER spent such an evening ... of heavenly love & happiness', Albert was a gentle lover and just to kiss him was a 'heavenly bliss'. 'He calls me Woman; I call him Man', mused the loved-up young queen, 'He treats me roughly, he scolds me, he gives me orders and I am happy that he does so.

Charles Kingsley and his wife Fanny, some years older than he, also revelled in a libidinous private world.

Charles, an historian, and preacher and canon at Westminster Abbey as well as a prolific author, wrote of the intensity of his desire for her: his hands so perfumed with her delicious limbs that he couldn't bring himself to wash off the scent, and how he spent almost his every moment thinking about her 'mysterious recesses of beauty', his heart sinking 'with a sweet faintness' and his blood tingling through every limb. They waited some years to marry (in 1844) and even then Charles asked her if she would consent to remaining a virgin for the first month of their married life so that they could achieve a more perfect delight when 'we lie naked in each other's arms, clasped together toying with each other's limbs, buried in each other's bodies, struggling, panting, dying for a moment'. Fanny, too, relished their carnal pleasures, writing to him that, 'We will undress and bathe ... you will take me up in your arms, will you not? And ... lay me down in bed ... and *come to me!*' Seven years after their marriage, Charles wrote to Fanny, Oh, those naked nights at Chelsea! When will they come again? I kiss both locks of hair every time I open my desk – but the little curly one seems to bring me nearer to you'.

So, for every well-recorded Victorian marriage which floundered in sexual fiasco, à la John Ruskin and Euphemia Gray's unconsummated union, there may have been a rapturous one. Take divorcée Emily Cavendish who seduced and later married the young virgin Count Gaston de la Rochefoucauld in 1870. Gaston, the infatuated boy-lover, declared that he had 'never kissed another woman ... you know too that nothing in you disgusts me ... I love and worship it all. It is a kind of madness'. His letters fervently listed their polymorphous activities: *cunnilingus*, *urinam bibendi*, *faeces devorandi*, and *delicias omnium corporis partium*. Emily, who washed herself too often for his liking, was forbidden soap and water more than once a day at most, for Gaston's 'tongue and saliva shall do the rest'. A different, but no less obsessive, rapture gripped Arthur Munby and his clandestine wife, Hannah Cullwick. They came from opposite ends of the Victorian class spectrum, but Arthur was a man much aroused by working women, compulsively collecting photographs of them and recording their experiences. Hannah became his willing 'slave' for fifty years, wearing a chain and bracelet to which her 'Massa' held the key. They had met on a London street in 1854 and their self-confessed 'peculiar love' revolved around Arthur's fetish about female strength, sweat, and dirt (Salirophilia is a sexual fetish that revolves around soiling the object of one's desire). Hannah was much the bigger and fleshier of the two and often carried him about the house, sat 'and nursed him ... Massa sits on me, feet and all on my knees'. She not only polished his boots for him, she lovingly licked them clean, 'she must be dirtier and coarser ... because she was *his*'. 'It's painfully delightful to suffer so much for love', wrote Hannah, and if ever her lover was cruel he would afterwards caress her, saying that 'whatever he did I should still be his slave'. Their powerful passion nurtured sexual and social sadism as well as Arthur's need for being worshipped and, frankly, coddled like a baby.

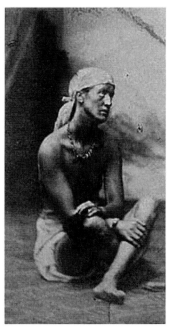

▲ Hannah Cullwick in 1862, dressed as a chimney sweep.

In America in the 1870s, Mabel Loomis Todd and David Todd were similarly enraptured, even reading his letters had 'truly a physical effect' on her. She wrote in her diary:

Every night he undressed me on the bright Turkey rug before the fire ... & loved me so!

Then, in the morning, he would carry her from the bed to the rug again, feeding her on figs and grapes. There was often 'a little Heaven just after dinner' when she would 'receive the precious fluid at least six or eight minutes after [her] highest point of enjoyment'. Even as they lusted after one another, Mabel, with David's complicity, took an older lover. Her husband encouraged her, taking vicarious erotic pleasure in her liaison, discreetly keeping out of the way when the lovers were upstairs together. David, after all, pleasured most of the female guests who visited their house and even seduced his daughter's friends when they were of an age.

Some late-Victorian doctors knew that sexuality was more than just biological: in a medical reference work of 1889, J. M. Duncan noted that even if a woman's ovaries were removed, her sexuality was not necessarily diminished. Still, the external sex organs were seen as more significant in determining a person's 'true' sex, and medico-legal reports on cases of 'hermaphrodism' were most concerned with fixing the sex of ambivalent individuals who formed a sort of loophole in an otherwise increasingly ordered taxonomy of sexual identities. In the adventurer Sir Richard Burton's translation of the *Kama Sūtra* (1883) there were 'two kinds of eunuchs or hermaphrodites; those who choose the role of men, and those who disguise themselves as women' (Alain Daniélou's translation of 1994 says, 'People of the third sex are of two kinds, according to whether their appearance is masculine or feminine'). In late-Victorian Britain, the *Kama Sūtra* was the only source for most people's knowledge of classical India – as if modern Western civilization was only known in Asia by the output of the American sex industry. Asia had become a site for the projection of Western erotic fantasies as opportunities for travel widened and cross-cultural ideas on sexuality spread: Victorian British men going abroad to do a spot of empire-building came into close contact with other ideas and activities and many took advantage of the perceived freedoms, joining in enthusiastically. Burton was a Vice-President of the Anthropological Society of London in the 1860s and also translated *The Book of a Thousand Nights and a Night, The Perfumed Garden*, and other erotic works. He poked Victorian sexual hypocrisy with the *Kama Sūtra's* unabashed and polymorphous sexuality.

Burton argued that 'the love of boys has its noble, sentimental side', and that the Platonists, followed later by the Sufis or Moslem Gnostics, 'held such affection, pure and ardent, to be the beau idéal which united in man's soul the creature with the Creator'. This pedarastic, Uranian love was said to be the most pure and beautiful in the world, 'passing as it does the love of women' in cleanliness, beauty and truth. Burton's wife was less impressed and destroyed much of her husband's work after his death, including that on pederasty; 'Why', she asked, 'did he wish the subject of unnatural crime to be so largely aired and expounded – he had such an unbounded contempt for the Vice and its votaries?'. In fact, Burton's interest dated at least from his posting to India in the 1840s where he wrote a report on male brothels (*lupanars*) in Karachi, and was suspected of 'participant observation'.

Poetic Uranian love emerged from Classical study and Hellenism as a justification for heavenly love between males, the *paiderastia* of ancient Greece, describing it as noble and intellectual, not frightening, disgusting or immoral. It offered 'truths' to modern men, a way to interpret and justify their own desires – they didn't have to think of themselves as necessarily homo- or heterosexual. Plato's *Banquet* was the 'most beautiful and perfect of all [these] works', according to Percy Bysshe Shelley when he translated it in 1818. Shelley's version wasn't published in his lifetime, mostly because he was worried about the propriety of its direct attitude to 'boy-love'. In early nineteenth-century England, men and boys were hanged for having sex with each other, though across the Channel the Napoleonic Code (established in 1804) stated that it was legal for males over the age of consent. However, French officials often ignored the law and saw pederasts and sodomites as a threat to public morals, thereby treating them harshly. Edgar Allan Poe considered Uranian love an 'elevating excitement of the soul', in his essay 'The Poetic Principle' (1850). But it was, he wrote, 'quite independent of that passion which is the intoxication of the Heart, or of that truth which is the satisfaction of the Reason. For in regard to passion, alas! its tendency is to degrade rather than to elevate the Soul'. Ronald Hyam, in *Empire and Sexuality: The British Experience*, debates the meaning of 'perversion', arguing that human sexual behaviour lies in variation rather than deviation, and that intention, attitude and consent are the important elements. A 'loving relationship between a man and a consenting boy, usually at or past the age of puberty…might become for later generations incomprehensible, misguided or illegal, but it is not from a theoretical point of view a perversion'.

Uranian verse embodied a longing for an attachment to a boy, usually from the lower-class, and it has been suggested that this sort of relationship relieved the older man of the rigours and responsibilities of a love affair with an intellectual equal, or that younger boys were sexually uninhibited at a time when women were more restrained and had too much to lose. It had a central role in upper-class homosexual subculture and included the poets John Addington Symonds, Lord Alfred Douglas, and the Rev E. E. Bradford, among others. In July 1914, the Uranians founded an official organization, The British Society for the Study of Sex Psychology, ostensibly to delve into all forms of sexual pathology and psychology. In reality it concentrated itself on pederasty, which they considered superior to the 'animal sexuality' between men and women, a stance that was openly and disastrously mocked as 'the higher sodomy'. *Water Cherubs*, written by the Uranian writer, Ralph Chubb in 1937, raised this sexuality to the realms of religious experience:

I choose the Boyish Body because it is the divine image & better than anything else expresses the whole mystery of life ... Love never harms, it blesses body & soul... everything in life without a single exception – from the Buttercup to the Sun, from the ... human babe to the unfolding World – is a sexual symbol of a Spiritual Fact.

Hostility to pederasty, now subsumed within paedophilia, continued to grow over the twentieth century.

Foucault credits the German neurologist and psychiatrist Westphal for naming homosexuality in his famous article of 1870 on 'contrary sexual sensations', though it was also used by the Hungarian, Károly M. Kertbeny, in 1869. Homosexuality appeared as a separate sexuality when sodomy, as a temporary aberration, metamorphosed into this new sexual identity, a 'hermaphrodism of the soul'. As it was medicalized it became a lesion, symptom, and dysfunction; a sexual identity as a psychiatric disorder. Homosexuality was, according to Burton, 'due sometimes to instinctive preference, sometimes to external conditions unfavourable to normal intercourse', and definitely a world-wide phenomenon, most usual in the 'Sotadic Zone' (which Burton named for the Greek poet Sotades) stretching from the Mediterranean, eastwards through the mountains of Western and Central Asia as well as the South Seas and the Americas (so 'geographical and climatic' rather than racial). In this zone there was 'a blending of the masculine and feminine temperaments, a crasis which elsewhere occurs only sporadically... one of the marvellous list of amorous vagaries which deserve, not prosecution but the pitiful care of the physician and the study of the psychologist'. This blending of sexuality was apparent in a crisis of masculinity in late nineteenth-century literature: in, for example, Rider Haggard's *She* (1886–7); Robert Louis Stevenson's *Dr Jekyll and Mr Hyde* (1886); in the life and writing of Oscar Wilde (1854-1900); and in J. M. Barrie's *Peter Pan* (1904).

Lesbianism, famously denied by Queen Victoria, was of less interest to the authorities than male homosexuality as it appeared to pose no threat to the status quo. According to Burton, 'the fact that homosexuality has been much more frequently noticed in men than in women does not imply that the latter are less addicted to it. For various reasons the sexual abnormalities of women have attracted much less attention, and moral opinion has generally taken little notice of them'. However, 'they' had been getting on with it all the time: Anne Lister (1791–1840), an educated woman of independent means, considered herself husband to M—, forsaking all others. Still she shared her fantasies of 'meeting a girl on Skircoat Moor, taking her into a shed there ... & being connected with her. Supposing myself in Men's clothes & having a penis'. When they came out in public, however, reactions were ugly: a specific line in Radclyffe Hall's *The Well of Loneliness* (1928) – 'and that night they were not divided' – was accused of inducing 'thoughts of a most impure character and would glorify the horrible tendency of lesbianism'. Male sexuality, whichever way it might lean, was still the more obviously powerful, at least in the West.

7

Sexuality and identity

I think rigid heterosexuality is a perversion of nature

Margaret Mead

The categorization of sexuality and its meaningful interpretation has led to something we are all now familiar with: the desire to enhance what we have 'discovered'. Synthetic hormones in particular brought an early promise of greater virility for both men and women. Hormones were 'sexed' by endocrinologists who arbitrarily bestowed sexual identity onto the chemicals they were synthesizing – and were later more than surprised to find that the testes of stallions contained five hundred times more oestrone than the ovaries of mares.

In France, Charles-Édouard Brown-Séquard had been experimenting on a rejuvenating elixir from the 1850s; the ingredients included macerated dog or guinea pig testicles. Monkey-gland operations were devised by Serge Voronoff in the 1920s – he had a monkey farm on the Italian Riviera. Much like cosmetic surgery used to be, this was an expensive and glamorous procedure and, like that aspect of the sex and beauty market, the practitioners held their patients in low esteem, even as they made high profits. A Viennese surgeon, Eugen Steinach, developed a rejuvenation operation (the bilateral vasectomy) and it was performed on, among other prominent middle-aged men, the Irish poet and statesman W. B. Yeats. Yeats was in his sixties and, allegedly, his work and libido were much revived; his surgeon was the Australian sexologist, Norman Haire, a liberal homosexual member of the British Society for the Study of Sex Psychology. In America, the novelist Gertrude Atherton, who associated Oscar Wilde with decadence and loss of virility, had her ovaries x-rayed to make her 'sparkling' again. Even thirty years later, the gynaecologist Robert Wilson, author of *Feminine Forever*

(1966), was arguing that post-menopausal women were redundant 'castrates'. A diminished sexuality had come to mean a diminished self.

Enjoying one's sexuality was the key, not only to a successful marriage, but to health and happiness. The West was beginning to discover this new 'truth' through books such as Marie Stopes' best-seller *Married Love* (published in 1918; by 1938 it had sold over 800,000 world-wide). A sex guidance and birth control pioneer, Stopes advocated understanding and mutual desire between husband and wife – an eroticization of marriage – even though her own was less than happy, and she was contemptuous of male doctors' attitudes to female sexuality. The intimate lives of the new breed of sexologists and psychologists were often fraught or unconventional, inspiring their work and advancing the movement towards increased knowledge, less prejudice, and greater freedoms for their educated middle-class peers and, eventually, for the lower classes. In 1929, Janet Chance established a birth control clinic in Kensington, London, and set up the first marriage guidance centre in Britain. By 1936 she had co-founded the Abortion Law Reform Association and believed that:

On the whole in England, sexual life is a poor thing. It is not happy; often it is wretched.

Women's sexual pleasure was supposedly derived less through orgasm or technique than through pleasing their husbands and fulfilling their wifely duty. Oral histories reveal that discussing or demanding their own sexual pleasure was perceived as selfish and, worryingly for the status quo, destabilizing.

Given this, the philosopher Bertrand Russell's *Marriage and Morals* (1929) was a highly controversial book – a rational look at sexuality and the often absurd rules that govern it. The book was aggressively denounced when it came out in America.

'Very few men or women who have had a conventional upbringing have learnt to feel decently about sex and marriage...Their education has taught them ... that sexual relations, even within marriage, are more or less disgusting, and that in propagating the species men are yielding to their animal nature while women are submitting to a painful duty. This attitude has made marriage unsatisfying to both to men and to women, and the lack of instinctive satisfaction has turned to cruelty masquerading as morality.'

This was 'Dynamite' according to the *New York Post*, while *Time Magazine* said it portrayed 'present-day laws and ideas about sex as an extraordinary potpourri obtained from savages, ascetics, Roman lawyers, Manichaean heretics, Teuton romanticists [all] based upon the idea of indissoluble connection between coition and conception, which is practically no longer true'. Enlightened sexual equality and contraception, so desperately needed, could be seen as either liberation or damnation.

Marie Stopes founded the first family planning clinic in the UK in 1921, in Holloway, North London. In the

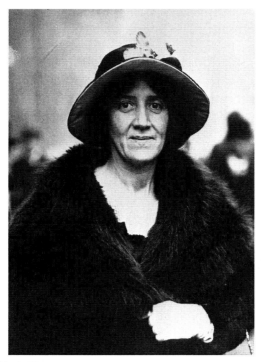

▲ Dr Marie Stopes
© *Bettmann/CORBIS*

following decade, five birth control societies were formed for 'children by choice, not chance'. Together, they became the National Birth Control Association in 1931, which in turn became the Family Planning Association (FPA) in 1939. By this time, sixty-five clinics were operating, though contraception was not provided for when the National Health Service was established in 1948. By 1952 the FPA was giving advice to women who were about be married and, eight years later, there were evening sessions for unmarried women, but only at the Marie Stopes Clinic in Whitfield Street, London. There remained very few clinics available for advice for unmarried women for another decade. In 1961 the pill was introduced in the UK (initially for married women only). Between 1962 and 1969, the number of UK users rose from approximately 50,000 to 1 million and this rapid take-up changed the relationship between sex and procreation, opening up new attitudes to sexuality. In 1967 the NHS (Family Planning) Act finally enabled the giving of birth control advice regardless of marital status The first vasectomy clinics opened in 1968, offering further options for family planning.

Condoms

The development of the rubber condom in the mid-nineteenth century and the contraceptive pill in the mid-twentieth were major shake-ups in sexual behaviours and attitudes. By the mid-nineteenth century, some London shops were selling condoms made of shapeless vulcanized rubber which could be washed and reused until they perished. By 1901 condoms had a fluid reservoir, and in 1912 latex ones were introduced. These were mass-produced and given to soldiers world-wide, mainly as a prophylactic against disease. At this time, the Americans were calling them 'Dreadnoughts', which was a British make of raincoat. Coloured condoms were manufactured in Japan in 1949; there have been customized ones since the 1960s, flavoured ones since the 1980s, and in 1994 the thin polyurethane condom hit the market.

The emergence of HIV and AIDS in the 1980s allowed condoms to be advertised on television and in print, and a report in

1999 found there was a leap in condom use to a world-wide demand of 24 billion a year, mainly to stop the spread of infection (in polyurethane, too, for those with latex allergy). A new generation of condoms is now being developed made of a composite mix of a new nano-material called graphene and an elastic polymer such as latex. It will be 'thinner, stronger, more stretchy, safer and, perhaps most importantly, more pleasurable'. A female condom, the Femidom, was launched in 1992 but never really caught on in developed countries. However, developing countries are increasingly being encouraged to use them, as these are the areas hardest hit by the HIV virus and AIDS.

Anxieties surrounding sexuality grew alongside the burgeoning openness and discussion. Miscegenation (marriage between different races) was a hot issue: in the late nineteenth and early twentieth centuries, some states in America enacted laws preventing marriage between whites and any 'Negro, Mulatto, or Mongolian', and there was hostility towards liaisons between whites and Indian and African-Americans. Fears regarding concepts such as purity, corruption, and slavery portrayed white women as deluded victims in sexual danger. They were given to understand that their safety and 'protection' depended on loyalty to their race. Eugenics was gaining purchase in the 1920s and 30s, and the declining birth rate of the white middle class was considered by some to be 'race suicide'; those lobbying for the sterilization of black and indigent women were equating sexuality with race and class for political and religious reasons.

Josephine Baker

An erotic dancer born in St Louis, Missouri (1906–75), Baker had to move to Europe to find acceptance and success. She sailed to France and made her name in Paris in La Revue Nègre with her uninhibited *Danse Sauvage*, dressed only in feathers. Most infamously, she starred at the Folies-Bergère Theatre in a skirt made of bananas: 'The rear end exists', she said, 'I see no reason to be ashamed of it, [but] it's true that there are rear ends so stupid, so pretentious, so insignificant, that they're only good for sitting on'. She was such a sensation, albeit exploiting the mythical excessive sexuality of the 'savage', that she stayed and became a French citizen.

Western cultural anthropologists such as Margaret Mead (an American contemporary of Josephine Baker) who lived and worked with the aboriginal populations of Australia, the Pacific Islands, the Americas, and Africa, argued over the meanings of sexuality. Their work was used in debates about slavery, colonialism, class, and the treatment of women and homosexuals. In the midst of the Jazz Age, when Western society was struggling with the perceived problems of pre-marital sex, abortion, illegitimacy, prostitution, adultery and divorce, Mead published *Coming of Age in Samoa* (1928) and got a remarkable reception – mainly because she reported the apparent sexual freedom of young, single people there. Their apparent 'promiscuity' was hedged around with behavioural codes, but they could experiment and 'prepare themselves for marriage'. Mead applauded this, arguing that women should have love, sexual pleasure, and careers. Her own life was unconventional: she had three husbands as well as male and female lovers.

Bertrand Russell had advocated trial marriages and a liberal approach to adultery, and argued that men and women should only consider themselves committed with the first pregnancy. In his book *Marriage and Morals*, he cited Polish-born Bronisław Malinowski's book, *The Sexual Life of Savages in North-Western Melanesia* (1929), as questioning conventional Western sexual mores.

> *The primary motive of sexual ethics as they have existed in Western civilization since pre-Christian times has been to secure that degree of female virtue without which the patriarchal family becomes impossible.*
>
> Bertrand Russell, Marriage and Morals

Male virtue, where it existed, was based in asceticism and, Russell believed, 'reinforced by female jealousy', exacerbated by emancipation. He believed women would prefer a system that allowed 'freedom to both sexes rather than imposing on men the restrictions' they had suffered. *Marriage and Morals* influenced the views of both Marie Stopes and Margaret Sanger, a birth control activist who had been arrested and jailed in 1916 for opening the first birth control clinic in Brooklyn, NY. She also allegedly had a 'rather bizarre and abnormal relationship' with Havelock Ellis who was also cited in Russell's book.

The Growth of Sexual Reassignment Surgery

In 1930s Britain, there were a series of Sunday newspaper stories about sex-change operations that added to the mass circulation of ideas about sexuality and sexual identity. The now defunct *News of the World* reported that a twenty-four-year-old woman, Doris Purcell was about to 'undergo a series of operations to have her sex changed to that of a man', though the language of the popular press was usually coy and euphemistic; they avoided terms such as 'intersexuality' or 'hermaphrodism'. Surgical techniques in plastic genito-surgery were advancing, as was the development of endocrinology. Another story told of Roberta Cowell, who had been a racing driver, Spitfire pilot and a prisoner of war, and was married with two daughters before she underwent gender-reassignment surgery in 1948. Her autobiography recounts her realization that she had been hiding 'what I knew deep down inside me though not consciously: my nature was essentially feminine and in some way my world was out of joint'. Psychoanalysis told her that her 'unconscious mind was predominantly female', and a Harley Street sexologist, who gave her a physical examination, noted prominent feminine sex characteristics. Reflecting the confused theories of the day, Roberta thought a 'series of emotional upsets' were the cause but that she also had a unique medical condition.

Despite some prurient interest, people who identified across genders were beginning to work with doctors to legitimize and make available sex-change procedures and, in doing so, they established the identity of transsexuality.

Wilhelm Reich, a pupil of Freud and a sexual evangelist, had been part of a movement for sexual reform in Berlin and Vienna which had been quashed by the Nazis, who believed it to be a corrupting Jewish conspiracy. He arrived in New York in August 1939 to an America steeped in sex (via Hollywood and advertising, for example) despite or because of its Puritan history. Reich had coined the term 'sexual revolution' in 1930, believing that true political revolution was only possible once sexual repression was brushed aside, and that Marxism and psychoanalysis together would mend the world. His book, *The Function of the Orgasm* (1927), argued that neurotics were suffering from a 'lack of full and repeated sexual satisfaction' and his orgone energy accumulator could restore them to health by improving their 'orgastic potency'. Sitting inside this wooden box lined with metal, Reich claimed that people were charged with orgone energy, a renewing life-force. Counter-culture figures such as Norman Mailer, J. D. Salinger, Allen Ginsberg, Jack Kerouac and William Burroughs all tried it out – the latter reporting spontaneous orgasm in his box. Reich, the instigator of 'a new cult of sex and anarchy', was soon under investigation by the FDA, imprisoned in 1957, and his books and remaining accumulators were burnt. He died of a heart attack in the Lewisberg Federal Penitentiary, eight months after being sentenced by the authorities who had ridiculed his ideas but nonetheless saw them as sufficiently dangerous to have him locked away.

Lullaby by W. H. Auden

Reich's *Function of the Orgasm* was published in 1940, the same year as W. H. Auden's poem *Lullaby*:

Lay your sleeping head, my love,

Human on my faithless arm;

Time and fevers burn away
Individual beauty from
Thoughtful children, and the grave
Proves the child ephemeral:
But in my arms till break of day
Let the living creature lie,
Mortal, guilty, but to me
The entirely beautiful.
Soul and body have no bounds:
To lovers as they lie upon
Her tolerant enchanted slope
In their ordinary swoon,
Grave the vision Venus sends
Of supernatural sympathy,
Universal love and hope;
While an abstract insight wakes
Among the glaciers and the rocks
The hermit's carnal ecstasy.
Certainty, fidelity
On the stroke of midnight pass
Like vibrations of a bell,
And fashionable madmen raise
Their pedantic boring cry:
Every farthing of the cost,

All the dreaded cards foretell,

Shall be paid, but from this night

Not a whisper, not a thought,

Not a kiss nor look be lost.

Beauty, midnight, vision dies:

Let the winds of dawn that blow

Softly round your dreaming head

Such a day of welcome show

Eye and knocking heart may bless,

Find the mortal world enough;

Noons of dryness find you fed

By the involuntary powers,

Nights of insult let you pass

Watched by every human love.

Bodies of knowledge about sexuality, from antiquity to the present day, have used cognate sciences such as zoology, anatomy, embryology and psychiatry, and by 1900 had shaped the discipline known as sexology. Alfred Kinsey was a professor of zoology at Indiana University and a specialist in wasps when he mixed his passions for collecting and taxonomy with the study of human sexuality. His questionnaires and statistics (plus, perhaps, some credulity in his subjects' veracity) led to the publication of *Sexual Behaviour in the Human Male* in 1948 and *Sexual Behaviour in the Human Female* in 1953, known as the Kinsey Reports. Revolutionary and controversial, the books on the much sex-surveyed American population revealed extensive faith in science – though Margaret Mead, for one, thought Kinsey had not paid enough attention to love. Heterosexuality was brought into focus through the classification of paraphilias, and 'facts' helped sexologists develop a concept of the norm and the abnormal, influencing attitudes towards sexuality. Even so, copies of the Kinsey Reports were seized by police, and four major publishers were prosecuted, three of them convicted. To see what sexologists considered the most extreme behaviours and desires is to know what society found most dangerous and frightening about sexuality.

William Masters and Virginia Johnson, who published *Human Sexual Response* (1966), did their research in the laboratory, using not personal interviews but direct observation. They recruited hundreds of couples, not all of them married, aged between eighteen and eighty-nine years, wired them up and filmed them. Masters and Johnson noted the stages of sexual response for both men and women, that the size of a penis is not linked to performance, that women can be multi-orgasmic, and that older people have sex, too. They also revealed that the female orgasm was clitoral, dismissing Freud's idea that it was either clitoral (immature) or vaginal (mature, elicited by men). Women's sexuality was no longer a reflection of men's sexuality. As their books sold out and the couple (who married in 1971) became celebrity favourites with the media, the language they used – such as clitoris, orgasm and masturbation – were suddenly, it seemed, released into the mainstream world. Cutting edge they may have been in the 1960s, but they were criticized in 1979 over their book *Homosexuality in Perspective* for arguing that gay men and women could have their 'sexual problems' treated and for suggesting cures. Shere Hite was a later critic, arguing that people needed to understand the 'cultural and personal construction of sexual experience to make the research relevant to sexual behavior outside the laboratory' – sex at home was not the same as sex in a lab. Nonetheless, medicine was still in the 'dark era' when it came to human sexuality, especially female sexuality, so when Masters and Johnson's findings came out they were a huge hit, despite the deliberately frosty scientific language. They were dispelling many previously-held myths and ushering in the sexual revolution.

Sexologists struggled against a tide of prurient and fearful antagonism, often religiously motivated. Even in 1942, Eustace Chesser of Harley Street, London, was prosecuted for obscenity over his 'plain guide to sex technique', *Love Without Fear*, despite it being written expressly for married couples (as practically all such volumes have by necessity purported to be). Chesser's ideas were a benevolent, if traditional, prelude to a new sexual revolution. In the 'normal sexual embrace', Chesser asserted, the wife 'submits', the husband 'takes' or 'possesses' her. Kissing was unconditionally recommended though, especially if 'lovers mutually explore and caress the inside of each other's mouths with their tongues as profoundly as possible, sometimes for hours', but lesbianism was summarily dismissed as being 'often due to practices indulged in at school'. Sexologists of the early and mid-twentieth century were a cuspate mix of taboo and liberality, a prelude to the hippy free-love movement of the 1960s, when sexual liberation would come around again, 'between the end of the "Chatterley" ban / And the Beatles' first LP'.

Lady Chatterley's Lover

D. H. Lawrence's novel was banned in Britain for more than thirty years because of its sexually explicit and controversial scenes. The novel tells of an adulterous relationship between a working-class man and a married upper-class woman, their affair crossing religious, political and sexual boundaries. When pirate copies were printed in America and sold at inflated prices, Lawrence quickly published *A Propos of 'Lady Chatterley's Lover'* (1929), to explain his beliefs: 'Obscenity', he wrote, 'only comes in when the mind despises and fears the body, and the body hates and resists the mind ... it is the mind we have to liberate'. The same year, police raided an exhibition of Lawrence's paintings and 'seized every canvas on which they could descry any wisp of pubic hair'. In 1959, The Obscene Publications Act allowed publishers to escape prosecution provided they could show a book was of literary merit; to this end Penguin printed 200,000 copies of the book at 3/6, putting it at easy reach of the masses. At the infamous trial that followed in 1960, Penguin were vindicated and sold 2 million copies over the next year alone. Mervyn Griffith-Jones, who led the prosecution, famously opened with the statement that the novel was not one 'you would even wish your wife or servants to read', thus revealing class distinctions, double standards, and a fine ignorance of popular culture and sexuality in the 1960s. The trial had major social and political consequences.

In the 1960s, human rights issues were fermenting in the public arena with the legalization of homosexuality and abortion, abolition of the death penalty, censorship, and reform of the divorce laws. Political and social change – witting and unwitting – were encapsulated by events such as the Profumo affair, a British political sex scandal of 1961–3. A government minister was brought down; the women involved, Christine Keeler and Mandy Rice-Davies, were vilified; and Steven Ward, brought to court to face trumped-up sexual charges, was demonized and committed suicide. British prurience and anxiety were projected onto Ward, 'the scapegoat who was sacrificed at the start of the low, libidinous decade'.

Abortion

In the UK, abortion was historically dealt with in church courts which allowed that abortion was acceptable before the 'quickening' (or the moment during pregnancy when the foetal movements can be first perceived). However, during the nineteenth and twentieth centuries a succession of laws were brought in which tightened up access to legal abortion. These laws did not, of course, prevent unwanted pregnancies or the demand for abortions, and many women were injured or died through resorting to back-street abortionists and or trying to do it themselves. In the early 1960s, 35,000 women a year needed NHS treatment following complications after enduring backstreet abortions. A further 10,000 women with their own or someone else's money could pay for terminations each year in West End clinics. Sex was a cash and class issue until the 1967 Abortion Act allowed abortion as long as the pregnancy 'has not exceeded its 24th week and that the continuance of the pregnancy would involve risk, greater than if the pregnancy were terminated, of injury to the physical or mental health of the pregnant woman or any existing children of her family'. After 24 weeks, abortion is allowed if there is risk to the life of the woman, evidence of severe foetal abnormality or risk of grave mental and physical injury to the woman.

In Northern Ireland, abortion can only be obtained if the woman's life is at risk and in some cases of foetal abnormality. Abortion was illegal in all US states by 1900 and remained so until 1973 (and the *Roe v. Wade* Supreme Court decision), yet women still had them. In 2013, senator Wendy Davis led a historic thirteen-hour long 'people's filibuster' to prevent a bill that could have stopped most women's access to abortion in Texas. She succeeded, and found support all over the world. In Australia, most people support pro-choice, regardless of religion or politics, yet there isn't universal and uniform access to abortion, possibly due to minority groups with hardline views and illiberal politicians – as Julia Gillard argued in her now famous 'misogyny speech'.

Influential, slow-burning ideas of sexual emancipation and political change, such as Reich's, took off in the upheaval of the mid-twentieth century. Although it has been argued that excitement and optimism leads people out of one set of restrictive ideas and into another, this period radically altered society's appreciation of different sexualities and freedoms. It was the 'second sexual revolution' according to *Time* (the first being the Jazz Age of the 1920s), but it came with a warning that the younger generation were 'adrift in a sea of permissiveness' and erroneously thinking that repression was a great evil and that sexuality was the province of science and not morals'. Eli Zaretsky, historian of psychoanalysis, has since argued that the new dawn of free love was commodified by the establishment, and a narcissistic 'sexualized dream world of mass consumption' has replaced the idealism.

8

New anxieties

Human beings have an inalienable right to invent themselves

Germaine Greer

The sexualization of Western society, through advertising and media, emphasizes youth and beauty at the expense of age, and dismisses the idea that sexuality extends throughout life. This trend arguably has greater implications for women, as menopause is commonly and historically seen as having a detrimental effect on female sexuality – yet this idea has never been supported by general population surveys. Recent research maintaining that women over forty might be having the best sex of their lives has proved predictably controversial. Despite taboos surrounding the sexuality of older people, studies confirm that sex can often remain an important part of life for men and women into their seventies, eighties, and beyond.

In the UK, government figures released in advance of World Health Day 2013 flagged up a change in HIV infection rates among older people: new cases of people over fifty years of age being infected through heterosexual sex rose from 239 in 2002 to 467 in 2012. The number of people aged fifteen to twenty-four infected with HIV through heterosexual contact in that same decade decreased from 483 in 2002 to 180 in 2012. The trend of older people being infected with HIV stretches across Europe, reflecting changes in social and sexual behaviour.

When HIV and AIDS emerged in the 1980s, the sexual revolution was shown to be a superficial phenomenon. Fear and prejudice were just below the surface, and its street name was the 'gay plague'. Predictions and responses were terrifying, the suffering was tragic. Today, the United Nations Joint Programme on HIV/AIDS (UNAIDS) says that the number of AIDS-related deaths is down, that record numbers of people are being treated, and new cases among children are down by more than half, but discrimination continues. AIDS-related deaths fell in the Caribbean by 50 per cent between 2001 and 2012 (down from 24,000 to 11,000); across Latin America there was a 37 per cent drop (from 82,000 to 52,000). In Europe and Central Asia, HIV infections have risen by 13 per cent (c.100,000 cases) since 2006, though across the continent less than 1 per cent of the population was HIV positive. AIDS-related deaths have risen in East Asia from 18,000 in 2001 to 41,000 in 2012. In sub-Saharan countries there were 1.2 million AIDS-related deaths and about 1.6 million people were infected across the continent in 2012, but the number of new cases of HIV was down 40 per cent. In the developed Middle East and North Africa, HIV cases rose by more than 50 per cent. A recent *Slate* magazine article on Africa, the epidemic's epicentre, argued that 'most of the measured improvements in AIDS in Africa are the result of cumulative, widespread behavior change' and are due to local African responses rather than any Western intervention. Local religious leaders are credited with curbing the spread of HIV through moral messages on fidelity and marriage – a trend that mirrors early patriarchal and punitive texts on sexuality from the first chapters in this book.

An American study on 'Sexual Activity and Function in Middle-aged and Older Women' (*Obstetrics and Gynaecology*, 2006) found that nearly three quarters of a diverse group of over 2,000 women aged between forty and sixty-nine were sexually active, and research by groups such as The Pennell Initiative for Women's Health have found that, at the menopause, 'women's sexual arousal or orgasm capacity actually increases'. A hundred years ago

Dr Heinrich Kisch wrote *The Sexual Life of Women*, marvelling that it was 'precisely in women of the climacteric age [that] there often exists a strong desire', though his influential contemporary, Dame Mary Scharlieb MD, thought it 'extremely pathetic to find women well on to fifty years of age who are apparently as keen on sexual enjoyment as a bride might be' (1915). Assumptions like these about the sexuality of older women have had serious implications for their health and status. Nineteenth-century doctors once recommended that women gave up sex completely when they hit forty, and prescribed drugs such as camphor to diminish sexual urges. Nowadays they prescribe drugs to enhance them.

If women do report a loss of sexuality, they may find themselves being treated to maintain a higher level of libido through drugs, despite an incompatibility with other aspects of their life, such as partners, work, children, elderly parents, status, and health. Pharmaceutical companies concentrating on Viagra for women have come up with 'female sexual dysfunctions' (FSDs) such as 'hypoactive sexual desire disorder', 'sexual aversion disorder', and 'female sexual arousal disorder', despite difficulties in defining 'libido' and 'dysfunction' which are based mainly on a narrow, 'genitally focused linear sequence model', i.e. desire, arousal and orgasm. A New York University psychiatrist calls FSD 'a textbook case of disease mongering', exploiting deep fears of suffering and death, and a decade ago the *British Medical Journal* suggested that it had been dreamed up by the pharmaceutical industry as a new market to exploit.

The OED defines 'libido' as 'a psychic drive or energy, particularly that associated with the sexual instinct, but also that inherent in other instinctive mental desires and drives'. Entrenched cultural expectations about female sexuality influence women's experience of libidinous changes, and moving the goalposts can radically change categorizations of what is 'normal' and what is 'dysfunctional'. Drug companies have been especially successful in America where there has been a heavily contested attempt to convince the public that 43 per cent of women in the US (50 per cent in the UK) have FSD. It is a terminally vague condition, preconceived and non-evidence based, defined by specialists who often turn out to be funded by the drug industry selling drugs to enhance sexuality: a robotic cruelty when they cannot arouse the mind. The mind, a powerful and often overwhelming force in arousal, is absent from diagnoses of FSD.

The jury is still out on whether the male menopause exists or not. In 1857, William Acton, in *The Functions and Disorders of the Reproductive Organs*, suggested men should expect sexual desire to fade because it was undignified and unnatural for the older gentleman, it was an unwelcome interruption on his journey to Christian perfection. He could, if he had the money, go to Brown-Séquard or Voronoff, or Marie Stopes who recommended electric shocks and marketed a device at her London clinic which conveniently plugged into any ordinary domestic light fitting – where electricity had been installed. Testosterone was isolated in 1935 and a cheap synthetic preparation became available as a wonder drug of all-round rejuvenation. In 1998, Viagra –

the name was coined from the words 'vigour' and 'niagra' – became the first oral medication for 'erectile dysfunction' to be approved by the United States Food and Drug Administration. The term 'erectile dysfunction' has replaced 'impotence' and shifted the emphasis from a perceived character flaw to a vascular problem. Pfizer, who manufactured the drug, saw their stock rise dramatically and sales topped 1 billion dollars within a year, giving a profit margin of 90 per cent. It was the fastest selling pharmaceutical in history. Sales bottomed out in 2000 and the focus now is on baby-boomers, though half of those who try it apparently do not renew their prescriptions. Casting doubt on male sexuality seems to be a far more delicate thing than humiliating women as unfeminine or sexually null.

Feminism had its own powerful impact on the baby-boomers and on present ideas of sexuality, one of the many influences variously suppressing or liberating, policing or cheering on difference. Sexual liberation, said to bring more 'joyous penetration', stood accused of phallocentricity and of ignoring female sexuality, homosexualities, and non-penetrative, non-genital sexualities. The much lauded 'healthy and true' heterosexual male libido, which was once the yardstick, is now just one facet in a kaleidoscope of sexualities. Feminism has kick-started many campaigns, both political and personal, on issues affecting women's health, status, and freedom. FORWARD (Foundation for Women's Health Research and Development) is 'an African Diaspora women-led UK-registered campaign and support charity dedicated to advancing and safeguarding the sexual and reproductive health and rights of African girls and women' working in the UK, Europe and Africa. Female Genital Mutilation (FGM) is one of their major causes, historically bound up as it is with complex social orders and traditional codes of behaviour relating to notions of female sexuality, purity and marriageability.

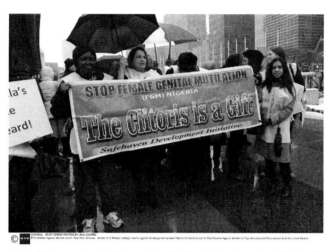

▲ End Violence Against Women March, New York, America – 08 March, 2013. Women holding a banner against female genital mutilation
REX/Sipa USA

FGM varies in severity, from the partial excision of the clitoris to its total removal plus that of the inner labia and the outer labia being sewn together (infibulation). The ritual affects the lives of women in many ways, aside from the obvious health risks, pain, and difficulties with sexual response, and there are intimations of being 'unclean', and 'immoral' if they are not cut. It is a practice with ancient precedents – it has been found in Egyptian mummies. The Victorian explorer Richard

Burton, recounting his travels in Africa and Asia, opined that female circumcision was necessary because the women were sexually voracious and too demanding for their circumcised men – they had to be modified to fit the dominant male desire. The World Health Organization (WHO) estimates that over 140 million women world-wide have suffered FGM, most commonly in northeast and west Africa, but also in the Arabian Peninsula and Indonesia. Something like a quarter of a million women in America have undergone FGM or are at risk of it, and in Britain the figure is about 66,000. The women are mostly from Africa, with a further 20,000 of their daughters also thought to be at risk. Many are illegally taken abroad for the ritual cutting, which is often done in secret and without anaesthetic. Some in Africa have accused anti-FGM campaigns of being just a new form of colonial and cultural interference and evidence of a decadent Western obsession with sex. But according to WHO, FGM is a 'pressing human rights issue and reliable evidence about its harmful effects, especially on reproductive outcomes, should contribute to the abandonment of the practice'.

Male Circumcision

This is the removal of the foreskin, practised mostly by Jews, Muslims, and in many African societies; the slitting of the foreskin is practised in some Polynesian cultures, and subincision, the slitting open of the urethra, is practised in addition to circumcision in some Australian aboriginal societies.

Like female circumcision it has been thought to curb the libido. In mid-twentieth-century America, male circumcision was almost universal and the prevailing rationale was that it prevented the spread of disease, especially cancer.

And now female genital cosmetic surgery (FGSC) is on the rise. This is non-medically indicated cosmetic surgical procedures which change the structure and appearance of healthy external and interior genitalia of women and girls. The NHS carried out 2,000 labial reductions – labiaplasty – in 2010 (but this is possibly just 'the tip of the iceberg' as private clinics do not have to record data). According to a joint report by the Royal College of Obstetricians and Gynaecologists (RCOG) and the British Society for Paediatric and Adolescent Gynaecology (BritSPAG), this is a five-fold increase in the past decade. These bodies are concerned about those who request labiaplasty for aesthetic reasons – especially as full development doesn't really occur before the age of eighteen – and, in extreme cases, whether this is an aspect of body dysmorphic disorder. They recommend that women and girls need to be made aware of the wide variation of genital appearance, that inaccurate advertising is rife, and that the pornography industry and popular media can give an unrealistic and narrow picture of what women and girls should look like or aspire to.

Popular culture, the movie industry and the inner world of fantasy have long since collided – 'In America sex is an obsession, in other parts of the world it is a fact', said Marlene Dietrich – and the open internet window on sexuality is a form of scopophilia itself, only new in that the degree of visibility has changed so much. Pornography on the web is seen as either the ruin of society or a vehicle for change; whichever way it is seen, it is highly profitable (like sexual dysfunction). It is now estimated that some 420 million pages of porn exist and 35 per cent of all downloads each month are from porn sites. Child pornography on the internet has grown alarmingly, and is said to be worth approximately $3 billion a year in the US alone. Violence as an aspect of sexuality is one of the major problems believed to be exacerbated by unfettered internet access, and is a factor often cited in courts of law by prosecution and defence, but it is also often viewed just as entertainment. A steady rise in consumer technology and the internet has arguably fuelled many new behavioural addictions – online porn addiction is increasingly prevalent and potentially distorting perceptions of sexuality – though clinical psychologists think we may reach a plateau as we begin to adjust to our relatively new technological environment. This concern could be seen as similar to the anxieties surrounding television in the 1950s and 60s and the way it was thought to be encouraging the ʻpermissive societyʼ – anxieties which spurred on campaigns such as the Christian social activist Mary Whitehouseʼs National Viewersʼ and Listenersʼ Association.

The mind is where sexuality is sculpted. It is is a fundamental erogenous zone, or, as Frank Zappa sang it:

What's the ugliest
Part of your body?
(My darling)...
I think it's your mind

9

Sexuality is as wide as the sea

Sexuality is the lyricism of the masses

Charles Baudelaire

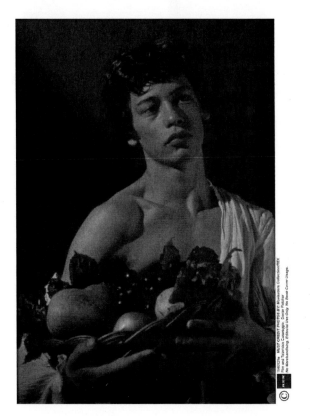

▲ Dexter Fletcher in Derek Jarman's 1986 film 'Caravaggio', a film about the life of Baroque painter Michelangelo Merisi da Caravaggio
REX/Moviestore Collection

More liberal attitudes to sexuality are gaining ground world-wide. In India, attitudes to lesbianism reflect the traditional roles of women in society and the family, ideas about obscenity and freedom of speech, the influence of the West, and ancient Indian erotic culture. Deepa Mehta's 1996 film, *Fire*, about a love affair between two women provoked protest and counter-protest, personified by the character Sita telling her lover Radha that, 'There is no word in our language to describe what we are or how we feel for each other'. *Bombay Dost*, launched in 1990, is India's first registered LGBT (Lesbian, Gay, Bisexual and Transgendered) magazine (the 20th anniversary issue featured Imran Khan talking about a kiss with actor Ranbir Kapoor on a TV show). The magazine has struggled in the past and, as a response to these difficulties, in 1994 organized the Humsafar Trust for self-identified gay men, MSM (men who have sex with men), transgenders, Hijras and LBTs to tackle HIV and provide education, prevention, care, support and treatment. Hijras are a religious sect of biological males who, over the last six hundred years, have dressed as and assumed the role of women; they don't consider themselves as either male or female, but as a third sex. A traditional minority in Indian society, they were invited to give blessings for fertility, but were ostracized with the arrival of the British. Many now live together in poverty, surviving through sex work, and have been hit hard by HIV and AIDS. The Humsafar Trust is also an umbrella organization for groups such as Umang – (for lesbian, bisexual women and LBTs) and Yaariyan (for young LGBT people). Attitudes are changing, but there remain dramatically contrasting cultural attitudes to sexuality around the world.

A similar umbrella organization, Transgender Europe (TGEU), was founded in 2005, and describes transgender people (or just 'trans people') as including those whose 'gender identity ... is different to the gender assigned at birth, and those who wish to portray their gender identity in a different way than the one they were assigned at birth.' An estimated 1 in 2,000 babies is born intersex or with a reproductive or sexual anatomy that does not fit typical definitions of male or female. Many 'feel they have to, or prefer or choose to, whether by clothing, accessories, cosmetics or body modification, present themselves differently to the expectations of the gender role assigned to them at birth. This includes, among many others, transsexual and transgender people, transvestites, cross dressers, no gender, [multigender], and genderqueer people, ... including interest and gender variant people who relate to or identify as any of the above'. TGEU is a member of the European Region of the International Lesbian, Gay, Bisexual, Trans & Intersex Association (ILGA-Europe), who work towards a world free of any discrimination due to sexual orientation, gender identity or gender expression, 'a world where the human rights of all are respected and everyone can live in equality and freedom'.

For intersex people – those born with genitalia not easily recognizable as obviously male or female, or born ambiguous and growing up differently to how gender was initially assigned – the question is whether a person must be one sex or the other, that physical sex is a binary affair, and that the apparently natural connection between your body and your gender is a given. Australia was the first country in the world, and Germany the first European country, to give a third option on birth certificates with the description 'indeterminate' under gender, allowing people to decide whether they want to be known as male or female later in life or to remain indeterminate. In 2012, Argentina passed a law allowing change of gender on birth certificates for transgender people. These changes are undeniable steps forward, but are still based on physical characteristics and the importance of perceived gender, even as the law moves to nullify any legal difference between them.

Advances in liberalization are, however, often accompanied by a backlash; it is a piecemeal process. As I finish this book, the Indian Supreme Court has reversed the landmark 2009 judgment that had decriminalized gay sex. Following a campaign by conservatives – including Muslim and Christian religious associations, a right-wing politician and a retired government official turned astrologist – they have reinstated a 153-year-old law passed under British rule, based on sixteenth-century English legislation, that defines 'carnal intercourse' between consenting adults of the same sex as 'unnatural' and punishable by up to ten years in jail. At the same time, the high court in Australia has ruled that the Australian Capital Territory (ACT) law cannot sit concurrently with the federal provision that marriage is between a man and a woman, and the entire ACT law 'is of no effect'. The country's first same-sex marriages were effectively annulled after just one week.

In Russia, President Putin has passed a number of anti-gay laws, including legislation that punishes people and groups that distribute information considered 'propaganda of non-traditional sexual relations'. Even as suicide numbers are on the rise, it has become illegal to offer information and support, and the country now has powers to arrest and detain foreign citizens believed to be gay, or 'pro-gay', provoking international concern and condemnation. There are more than seventy-five countries world-wide where homosexuality is still criminalized. In Europe, Turkish-occupied northern Cyprus is the only place in Europe where it remains illegal, but The Human Dignity Trust has filed a suit at the European Court of Human Rights, and looks likely to succeed. The Prime Minister of Trinidad and Tobago has said she wants to repeal laws that ban homosexuality, as has Jamaica's Prime Minister, Portia Simpson Miller and, in Malawi in 2012, the President, Joyce Banda, announced that laws criminalizing homosexuality would be quashed. Brazil now has full legal equality for different sexualities, but is experiencing a backlash of anti-gay crime – a gay person is murdered every thirty-six hours – and a religious and conservative right movement is now attempting to stop anti-homophobic laws and education.

There are still thirty-eight African countries where homosexuality is illegal – President Mugabe of Zimbabwe has said that he will never accept homosexuality, and that gay people are 'worse than pigs, goats and birds', while in Cameroon, Uganda, and Nigeria anti-gay laws are becoming ever more draconian. In Iran, homosexuality is punishable by death and the official line is that it is 'an illness that should be cured'. This idea of cure exists in America too, with a religious basis often backed by spurious science: the National Association for Research & Therapy of Homosexuality (NARTH) was founded in 1992 to offer various regimens towards a 'cure'. It was launched as a response to professional organizations, including the American Psychiatric Association who, NARTH maintains, had 'totally stifled the scientific inquiry that would be necessary to stimulate a discussion' about homosexuality. Their website suggests that what they call the 'homosexual revolution' is just 'a hint of the shape of things to come. If religious liberty means anything, it means the right to teach and practice biblical morality. Once this is forbidden, religious liberty is reduced to ashes. When', they ask, 'will America's Christians smell the smoke?' If it is impolitic to suggest that homosexuality is a disease or moral insanity, religion on the whole still sees it as a sin that must be vanquished, and it remains enshrined in law in many countries.

While the repressive McCarthy period of late-1940s to mid-1950s America was raging, when the FBI was seeking out subversive behaviour and homosexuality was demonized as both a crime and a disease, the psychologist Evelyn Hooker published 'The adjustment of the male overt homosexual' (1957). Her research had been encouraged by a gay friend and it revealed that there was no discernible psychological difference between heterosexual and homosexual men, debunking popular myths and leading to significant changes in the treatment of homosexuals. Hooker's study was a major part of the campaign which eventually led to the American Psychiatric Association removing homosexuality from the *Diagnostic and Statistical Manual of Mental Disorders* (DSM) in 1973 where it had been listed as a sociopathic personality disorder. Two years later, the American Psychological Association stated that, 'homosexuality per se implies no impairment in judgment, reliability or general social and vocational capabilities, [medicine should] take the lead in removing the stigma of mental illness long associated with homosexual orientation'. Homophobia is still with us though. A disproportionate number of homeless teenagers in America are LGBT, and their suicide rate is high. Norms, behaviours and mores may change, but stereotypes are harder to shift and it can be dangerous to challenge them.

In the UK in the 1960s, Leo Abse MP and Lord Arran, referring to the Wolfenden Report of 1957, which had been rejected by the Conservative government, put forward proposals to deal with the law on homosexuality. The Sexual Offences Act (1967) eventually decriminalized homosexual acts in private between two men in England, but they had to be over twenty-one. It wasn't until 1980 that this happened in Scotland, or 1982 for Northern Ireland, and it was still illegal in the armed forces and the navy until 2000. This legislation followed a period during the 1950s when increasing numbers of men were being prosecuted.

Wolfenden Report, 1957

'It is not, in our view, the function of the law to intervene in the private lives of citizens, or to seek to enforce any particular pattern of behaviour, further than is necessary to carry out the purposes we have outlined ... homosexual behaviour between consenting adults in private should no longer be a criminal offence'

For most of the twentieth century the label 'queer' was one of too many derogatory terms given to gay men and lesbians but in 1990, Queer Nation, founded in New York by AIDS activists to protest against violence and prejudice against LGBTs, began to rehabilitate the word to show some of the variability and possibility in a more fluid sexual world: 'We're Here. We're Queer. Get Used To It'. Gay and lesbian identity politics became more and more visible towards the end of the century, especially after the violence between police and gays at the Stonewall Inn in New York in 1969, and the idea of sexual identities began to move out of medical language and into that of civil rights. For many, Stonewall heralded the beginning of the gay movement.

Understand that sexuality is as wide as the sea ... that your morality is not law ... that we are you. Understand that if we decide to have sex whether safe, safer, or unsafe, it is our decision and you have no rights in our lovemaking.

Derek Jarman (1942–1994)

Just as there are many attitudes towards homosexuality, so are there plenty of theories on why someone is gay – and we might wonder why finding a 'cause' is so important. Religion on the whole has considered it a sin, medicine as a disease, and the state as a subversion. Ideas include the possibility that it is a 'perverse' choice, or that the young are seduced into it by the old, that they have smothering mothers or absent and aloof fathers, traumatic early heterosexual experiences or it is in our genes. Present-day Darwinian philosophy influences the study of genetics, gender and sexuality in that there is a conflict between the ideas of gender as a social construct and gender as something biologically constructed or determined. Natural selection, it is argued, doesn't work through culture, rather reproduction demands dividing into two parts: males competing and females caring for offspring. The idea of genes can be disturbing because of its determinism and denial of free will, and many people, unsurprisingly including feminists and lesbians, object to the idea that sexuality can be seen as so bluntly biological and not cultural. Epigenetics has become something of an antidote to genetic determinism, offering the possibility that our genetic code is a rough guide that can change. Genes respond to the environment, and one way of doing it is to switch themselves on and off with different cues, colder temperatures, for example, and X chromosome inactivation (X-inactivation was discovered in 1961 by British scientist Mary Lyon). Women have two X chromosomes, whereas men have one; one having switched off after about twelve weeks of embryonic development. All the genes are still there, but in males only half of them are necessary. The process is shaped by hormones, and it's not just the sex organs, but the brain and psychology of the new child that are being shaped too, including sexual orientation and preference.

Identical male twins sometimes differ – one may be born with homosexual preferences and the other not – yet they have the same genes, so hormones shaped them differently to each other because of levels and timing: same genes, different outcome. Neuroscientist Simon LeVay was a pioneer in sexual orientation in the early 1990s, and his book, *Gay, Straight, and the Reason Why: The Science of Sexual Orientation* (2011), gives an overview of the recent arguments in neuroscience, endocrinology, genetics and cognitive psychology. He exposes cross-cultural contradictions in understanding and belief and shows that searching for a 'cause' of homosexuality is altogether too simplistic. Rather, he argues for a 'spectra of gender diversity', and that the common notion that gender-based differences (the female/male divide) that drive our sexual orientation is narrow and rigid. LeVay suggests that instead of thinking about sexuality in terms of same-sex and opposite-sex attraction, we think in terms of gynephilia (attraction to females) and androphilia (attraction to males), meaning that stigma, labelling and psychological suffering would be lessened. He argues that we need to think about sexuality in other ways, and that cultural forces have greatly influenced how it has been expressed in different societies and across time. There are limits, he says, 'to what we may hope to explain with biological ideas'. American writer, self-identified lesbian femme and a founder of the Lesbian Sex Mafia set up in 1981 in New York, Dorothy Allison, has argued that, 'Class, race, sexuality, gender and all other categories by which we categorize and dismiss each other need to be excavated from the inside'.

After loss of identity, the most potent modern terror, is loss of sexuality, or, as Descartes didn't say, "I fuck therefore I am".

Jeanette Winterson, *Art & Lies: A Piece for Three Voices and a Bawd* (1996)

Sexuality is so fundamental to human experience, so compelling and so powerful in its presence or apparent absence that, alongside the jouissance, it has always provoked dissension, disruption, and control. It would be astonishingly arrogant to presume that there is a right way for people to experience, understand or express their sexuality. Over the centuries we have lived under all manner of socially sanctioned ideas, policies, and behaviours – some immensely complex – and sexuality has always tempted commentators into trying to describe and define it; poets, artists, doctors, scientists, novelists, lawyers, philosophers, *et al.* This short book has attempted this seemingly unlimited task also, or at the very least it has scratched the surface of their efforts, prejudices and desires for change. The American author, poet, and activist, Alice Walker, has said that 'Sexuality is one of the ways that we become enlightened, actually, because it leads us to self-knowledge'. Until it is described and discussed, its language and symbols explored, sexuality can seem very chaotic. Sexuality has always been tied, as Foucault remarked, to devices of power, and perhaps our recent politicization is just as manacled an approach as were the early church courts, medico-moral regulation, and the Victorian drive for categorization, wherein desire and identity were fused. We can't look at sexuality in isolation because it is intertwined with history, culture, class and race, with all of our social interactions and different ideas and behaviours. Today, sexuality seems to have less to do with biological gender and what we do with our genitals than with self-definition and satisfaction. Where, from the authoritarian descriptive and prescriptive to the personally diverse and transgressive, is the consensus? Can there be one and has there ever been one?

This 100 ideas section gives ways you can explore the subject in more depth. It's much more than just the usual reading list.

13 Novels

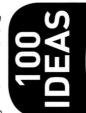

Leopold von Sacher-Masoch, *Venus in Furs* (1870) – this Austrian writer inspired the clinical category of 'masochism'.

Pauline Reage, *Story of O* (1954) – a novel of dominance and submission. Reage was the pseudonym of an intellectual and holder of the Légion d'Honneur, called Dominique Aury who had written the book at the age of 47 but not revealed her identity until she was 86.

Radclyffe Hall, *The Well of Loneliness* (1928) – a lesbian novel banned after official medical advice that it would encourage female homosexuality and lead to 'a social and national disaster'.

Rita Mae Brown, *Rubyfruit Jungle* (1973) - an American coming-of-age autobiographical novel; the term 'rubyfruit jungle' is slang for female genitalia.

Henry Miller, *Tropic of Cancer* (1934) – US censors suppressed this book until 1961. It has been described as 'a great, bloody sprawl of a book, an assault on the taste, the patience and the expectations of even the most adventurous of readers'.

John Updike, *Couples* (1968) – a novel about the life and sexual odyssey of a software designer. It was attacked for its 'preoccupation with small-town adultery'.

Lynne Reid Banks, *The L-Shaped Room* (1960) - an unmarried pregnant woman is thrown out by her father and befriended by a black neighbour and a Jewish writer, all of them outsiders in 1960s London.

Anaïs Nin, *Delta of Venus* (written 1940s, published posthumously 1977) – an anthology of erotic short-stories.

John Cleland, *Fanny Hill: or, the Memoirs of a Woman of Pleasure* (1748-9) – Cleland's novel, an early example of erotic fiction, tells the story of Fanny Hill from village girl to London prostitute and marriage.

Virginia Woolf, *Orlando: A Biography* (1928) – the 'longest love letter in the world', from Woolf to Vita Sackville-West. Orlando plays with time and gender.

A M Homes, *The End of Alice* (1997) – the story of a correspondence between a convicted paedophile and murderer and a young woman whom he comes to confuse with his original victim.

Philip Roth, *Portnoy's Complaint* (1969) – the story of sex-obsessed Alexander Portnoy which the New Yorker described as 'one of the dirtiest books ever published'. The guilt-ridden monologue of a young Jewish man in the 1960s it explores culture through sexuality. It is also very funny.

William S Burroughs, *Naked Lunch* (1959) – a trawl through sexual obsession and the human condition, this book has been described as 'an absolutely devastating ridicule of all that is false, primitive, and vicious in current American life'.

6 Pieces of music

'Je t'aime... moi non plus', Serge Gainsbourg (1969)

'Relax (Don't Do It)', Frankie Goes to Hollywood (1983)

'Salome', Richard Strauss (1905)

'Come Again, sweet love doth now invite', John Dowland (1597)

'Wreck a Buddy', The Soul Sisters (1969)

'Lover Man', Billie Holiday (1951)

10 political sex scandals

John Profumo, 1963 - Secretary of State for War in the British Government had an affair with Christine Keeler, described as a 'showgirl', and lied about it to the House of Commons. Keeler had also slept with Eugene Ivanov, the naval attache at the Soviet Embassy. The scape-goat was Stephen Ward, another friend of Keeler's, who killed himself in the aftermath.

Jeremy Thorpe, 1976 – Norman Scott alleged that he had had an affair with Thorpe in the early 1960s and that the politician and leader of the Liberal Party had threatened him. Thorpe was acquitted of the charge of conspiracy to murder.

Dominic Strauss-Kahn, 2011 – the former International Monetary Fund leader was accused by a New York hotel maid of sexual assault. His political career collapsed amid further revelations of his dealings with women in Europe, too.

Yoon Chang-yung, 2013 – a former presidential spokesman of South Korea, he was fired following a sexual assault on a female intern at the Korean Embassy to the US.

Silvio Berlusconi – years of allegations of sex scandals, as well as political corruption, finally ended with the Italian ex-prime minister's conviction of tax fraud in 2013. His sentence for having sex with an under-age girl and his abuse of power is currently being appealed.

Bill Clinton, 1998 – the American president had an affair with an intern, Monica Lewinsky, but stated that he did 'not have sexual relations' with her. He was impeached by the US House of Representatives in 1998.

Nils Quensel, 1951 – the Swedish Minister of Ecclesiastic Affairs was forced to resign over the sexual abuse of boys and a cover-up.

David Petraeus, 2012 – Retired Army Gen. David Petraeus resigned as CIA director after an FBI investigation revealed he'd had an extramarital affair and that his lover may have had inappropriate access to classified information.

Jacob Zuma, 2005 – charged and acquitted of the rape of an HIV-positive woman but strongly criticised for his ignorance of HIV-AIDS when his country is facing an epidemic. He was re-elected President of South Africa in the 2014 elections.

Moshe Katsav, 2010 – former Israeli president convicted of rape and other sexual offences towards more than three of his employees.

10 Artists

Frida Kahlo (1907–1954)

Katsushika Hokusai (1760–1849)

Marcantonio Raimondi (1480–1527)

Aubrey Beardsley (1872–1898)

Yayoi Kusama (1922–)

Tracey Emin (1963–)

Henri de Toulouse-Lautrec (1864–1901)

Peter Paul Rubens (1577–1640)

William Holman Hunt (1827–1910)

Robert Mapplethorpe (1946–1989)

11 Websites

http://www.bombaydost.co.in

http://www.forwarduk.org.uk/key-issues/fgm

http://www.equalitynow.org

http://www.dofeve.org

http://www.ilga-europe.org

http://www.thestranger.com/seattle/Savage Love?oid=
    18144030

http://www.beaumontsociety.org.uk

http://www.thetrevorproject.org

http://www.asexuality.org

http://www.mind.org.uk/information-support/guides-to-
    support-and-services/sexuality-and-mental-health/#.
    UpXq56W61rc

http://www.pinkstinks.co.uk

11 Films and plays

Fellini Satyricon, Frederico Fellini (1969)

Milk, Gus Van Sant (2008)

Fire, Deepa Mehta (1996)

Saturday Night, Sunday Morning, Karel Reisz (1960)

The Killing of Sister George, Frank Marcus (1964)

Staircase, Charles Dyer (1966)

Hedwig and the Angry Inch, John Cameron Mitchell (2001)

A Streetcar Named Desire, Tennessee Williams (1947)

Last Tango in Paris, Bernardo Bertolucci (1972)

La Cage aux Folles, Jean Poiret (1973)

Ghosts, Henrik Ibsen (1882)

11 Poems

Philip Larkin (1922–1985) *Annus Mirabilis*

Catullus (c.84–54 BCE) *Catullus 5*

Andrew Marvell (1621–1678) *To His Coy Mistress*

ee cummings (1894–1962) *somewhere i have never travelled, gladly beyond*

John Donne (1572–1631) *The Flea*

Maya Angelou (1928–2014) *Phenomenal Woman*

Aphra Behn (1640–1689) *The Disappointment*

Sharon Olds (1942–) *After Making Love in Winter*

Sarojini Naidu (1879–1949) *Suttee*

Robert Browning (1812–1889) *Porphyria's Lover*

Allen Ginsberg, (1926–1997) *Howl*

10 Classic texts

Shere Hite, *The New Hite Report* (2000)

Havelock Ellis, *Studies in the Psychology of Sex* (1897–1928), seven volumes.

Masters and Johnson, *Human Sexual Response* (1966)

Alfred Kinsey, *Sexual Behavior in the Human Male* (1948), and *Sexual Behavior in the Human Female* (1953)

Simone de Beauvoir, *The Second Sex* (1949)

Germaine Greer, *The Female Eunuch* (1970)

Bertrand Russell, *Marriage and Morals* (1929)

Michel Foucault, *The History of Sexuality* (three volumes, 1976–84)

Wilhelm Reich, *The Function of the Orgasm* (1927)

Oz magazine (1963–69 in Sydney, Australia and 1967–73 in London)

12 Quotes

Shakespeare, *Macbeth*, 'It provokes the desire, but it takes away the performance; therefore much drink may be said to be an equivocator with lechery: it makes him and it mars him', (first performance 1611).

John Garfield's *Wandering Whore (1660s)*, Julietta: 'He that thinks I had my Maiden head after thirteen, has had a knock in the Cradle'.

Hijra rights slogan C21, 'You don't need genitals for politics, you need brains and integrity'.

Philip Roth (1981) 'These days, when sexuality is no longer taboo, mere description, mere sexual confession, has become noticeably boring'.

Shere Hite, 'Anything over three people constitutes a group, anything over seven people an orgy'.

Muriel Spark, *The Prime of Miss Jean Brodie* (1961), 'One's prime is elusive. You little girls, when you grow up, must be alert to recognise your prime at whatever time of your life it may occur'.

E. M. Forster, 1928, 'My defence at any Last Judgement would be, "I was trying to connect up and use all the fragments I was born with".'

Savonarola, (1494) 'Abandon, I tell you, your concubines and your beardless youths. Abandon, I say, that unspeakable vice, abandon that abominable vice that has brought God's wrath upon you, or else: woe, woe to you!'.

Marlon Brando, 1975, 'Like the vast majority of men I've had several homosexual experiences and I'm not remotely ashamed of it'.

Mae West, 'Between two evils, I always pick the one I never tried before'.

Germaine Greer, 'Freud is the father of psychoanalysis. It had no mother'.

Mahatma Gandhi, 'You must be the change you wish to see in the world'.

5 Festivals

New Orleans Burlesque Festival, Louisiana USA

German Fetish Ball Weekend, Berlin, Germany

Sexy International Film Festival, Melbourne, Australia

Kinky Salon, Copenhagen, Denmark and Global

Phallus, Tyrnavos, Greece

Sources and Further Reading

Abelard, Peter and Heloise *Forbidden Fruit: From the letters of Abelard and Heloise*. Translated by Betty Radice. Revised by M. T. Clanchy (Penguin, 2007)

Appignanesi, Lisa, *Mad, Bad and Sad: A history of women and the mind doctors from 1800 to the present* (Virago, 2008)

Berkowitz, Eric, *Sex and Punishment: 4000 years of judging desire* (The Westbourne Press, 2013)

Bertholet, Ferry M., *Concubines and Courtesans : Women in Chinese erotic art* (Prestel, 2011)

Brown, Kevin, *The Pox: The life and near death of a very social disease* (Sutton, 2006)

Dabhoiwala, Faramerz, *The Origins of Sex: A history of the first sexual revolution* (Allen Lane, 2012)

de Botton, Alain, *How to Think More about Sex* (Macmillan, 2012)

Fang Fu Ruan, *Sex in China: Studies in sexology in Chinese culture* (Plenum Press, 1994)

Fisher, Kate and Toulalan, Sarah, eds., *Bodies, Sex and Desire from the Renaissance to the Present* (Palgrave Macmillan, 2011)

Foucault, Michel and Hurley, Robert *The History of Sexuality, Vol. 1: An introduction* (Penguin, 1979)

Foucault, Michel and Hurley, Robert *The History of Sexuality, Vol.2: The Use of Pleasure* (Viking, 1986)

Gibson, R., Green, S. and Sharrock, A., eds., *The Art of Love: Bimillenial essays on Ovid's Ars Amatoria and Remedis Amoris* (OUP, 2007)

Higgins, Patrick, ed., *A Queer Reader* (Fourth Estate Ltd, 1993)

Jolan Chang, *The Tao of Love and Sex: The ancient Chinese way to ecstasy* (Wildwood House Ltd., 1977)

Jütte, Robert, *Contraception, A History* (Polity Press, 2008)

Krysmanski, Bernd W., *Hogarth's Hidden Parts: Satiric allusion, erotic wit, blasphemous bawdiness and dark humour in eighteenth-century English art* (Olms, 2012)

Laqueur, Thomas, *Making Sex: Body and gender from the Greeks to Freud* (Harvard University Press, 1990)

Laqueur, Thomas, *Solitary Sex: A cultural history of masturbation* (NY: Zone, c2003)

LeVay, Simon, *Gay, Straight, and the Reason Why: The science of sexual orientation* (OUP, 2011)

Lyons, Andrew P. and Lyons, Harriet D., eds., *Sexualities in Anthropology: A reader* (Wiley-Blackwell, 2011)

Moore, Lisa Lynne, 'Queer gardens: Mary Delany's flowers and friendships' in *Eighteenth-Century Studies*, 39, No.1, Fall 2005, 49–70

Myerowitz, Molly, *Ovid's Game of Love* (Wayne State University Press, 1985)

Porter, R. and Teich, M., eds., *Sexual Knowledge, Sexual Science: The history of attitudes to sexuality* (Cambridge University Press, 1994)

Reis, Elizabeth, ed., *American Sexual Histories* (Wiley-Blackwell, 2012)

Rocha, Leon Antonio, 'The way of sex: Joseph Needham and Jolan Chang' in *Studies in History and Philosophy of Biological and Biomedical Sciences* 43 (2012) 611-626.

Rousseau, George, *Children and Sexuality from the Greeks to the Great War* (Palgrave Macmillan, 2012)

Rusbridger, Alan, *A Concise History of the Sex Manual* (Faber and Faber, 1986)

Speller, Lizzie, *The Illustrated Book of Orgies: A reflection on the beauty in numbers* (London: The Erotic Print Society, 2000)

Szreter, Simon, and Fisher, Kate, *Sex Before the Sexual Revolution: Intimate life in England 1918–1963* (CUP, 2010)

Thiher, Allen, *Revels in Madness: Insanity in medicine and literature* (University of Michigan Press, 2004)

Turner, Christopher, *Adventures in the Orgasmatron: Wilhelm Reich and the invention of sex* (Fourth Estate Ltd, 2011)

Turner, James Grantham, *Schooling Sex: Libertine literature and erotic education in Italy, France, and England 1534–1685* (OUP, 2003)

Vanita, Ruth, ed., *Queering India: Same-Sex Love and Eroticism in Indian Culture and Society* (Routledge, 2002)

Weston, Kath, *Long Slow Burn: Sexuality and Social Science* (Routledge, 1998)

Wilson, G. and Rahman, Q., *Born Gay: Psychobiology of sex orientation* (Peter Owen, 2008)

Acknowledgements

George Miller

Sam Richardson

Elizabeth Speller

Michael Bywater

Katy Foxcroft

Chella Adgopul

Nikki Zeeman

Index

Page numbers in italics refer to illustrations

aborigine 92, 112
abortion 101–2
Abortion Law Reform Association 87
Abse, Leo 124
Acton, William 56–7, 109
addiction
  online porn 114
  sex 68–9
Africa 122
age of consent 51–3
AIDS 90–1, 106–7
Akin, Todd 56
alcohol 14, 141
Allbutt, T. C. 67
Allison, Dorothy 127
Amakasu Incident 59
American Psychiatric Association 123
American Psychological Association
  123–4
An Essay on the Principle of Population
  44
*Ancient and Modern Pederasty
  Investigated and Exemplify'd* 45
androphilia 127
Anthropologia (Haworth) 16, 18
Aristotle's Masterpiece 33, 41
Ars Amatoria (Ovid) 13–4
art *see* erotic art
*Art & Lies: A Piece for Three Voices and
  a Bawd* 128
artists 26, 49, 136
Atherton, Gertrude 86
Auden, W. H. 95
Augustinian ideology 22–3
Augustine of Hippo 22
Augustus, Emperor 14
Australia 102, 121

Baartman, Saartjie 62–3, *63*
Baker Brown, Isaac 67
Baker, Josephine 92
Banda, Joyce 122
Banquet (Plato) 12, 80
Barrie, J. M. 83
Baudelaire, Charles 37, 117
Beardsley, Aubrey 49
Beethoven 37
Behn, Aphra 39
Bentham, Jeremy 9
Berlusconi, Silvio 134
birth control clinics 87, 88–90, 93
Blake, William 59
Boccaccio 26
Bombay Dost 119
Book of the City of Ladies 25
Book of a Thousand Nights and a Night
  79
Book of the Treasury of Ladies 25
Boswell, James 37, 48
Botero, Fernando 5
Bradford, Rev E. E. 81
Brando, Marlon 141
British Society for the Study of Sex
  Psychology 81, 86
Brown, Rita Mae 132
Brown-Séquard, Charles-Édouard 86
Buddhism 11
Burroughs, William 95, 133
Burton, Richard 13, 78–9, 82, 83, 111–2
Butler, Josephine 38, 56

Cannon, Thomas 45, 46
Canterbury Tales 26
'Caravaggio' (film) *118*
Casanova 37, 49–50

Castlehaven, Mervyn Touchet, Earl of 38
catamites 10
Cavendish, Emily 75–6
censorship
    of *Lady Chatterley's Lover* 100–1
    of Ovid 14
Chance, Janet 87
Chang-yung, Yoon 134
Chaucer, Geoffrey 21, 26
Chesser, Eustace 99
child pornography 114
childhood sexuality 50–3, 58
China
    Neo-Confucianist puritans 11
    Taoist writings (c.2000 bce) 10–1
Christianity
    on non-procreative sex 23
    sex linked with sin 22–3
Chubb, Ralph 81
Church, regulation of sexuality by
    26, 38–9
Churchill, Randolph 37
circumcision
    male 112–3
    see also female genital mutilation
Cleland, John 44–5, 132
Clinton, Bill 134
clitoridectomy 67, 111–2
clitoris 30, 31, 98
Coming of Age in Samoa 92
concupiscence 18, 26
condoms 34–5, 90–1
'Conjugal Lewdness or, Matrimonial
    Whoredom' 44
contraception
    in 18th cent. 44, 50
    condoms 34–5, 90–1
    on the NHS 88, 89
    the pill 90
    word first used 44
    see also family planning clinics

Couples 132
Cullwick, Hannah 76, *77*
Culpeper, Nicholas 31
Cuvier, Georges 63

Darío, Rubén 5
Darwinianism 58, 126
de Pizan, Christine 25
Decameron, The (Boccaccio)
    26
Defoe, Daniel 44
Delaney, Mary 48
Delta of Venus 132
*Diagnostic and Statistical Manual of
    Mental Disorders (DSM)* 65,
    123
Diderot, Denis 33, 47
Dietrich, Marlene 113–4
'discursive explosion' 4
diseases, sexual 34–8
Don Juanism 68–9
Douglas, Lord Alfred 81
Dr Jekyll and Mr Hyde 83
Du Laurens, André 18
Duncan, J. M. 78

East of Eden (Steinbeck) 1
Eastern culture
    11th-15th cent. 27–8
    Victorian sexuality and 78–9
    see also China; India
eggs, women's 31
ejaculation, draining the *qi* 10
Ellis, Havelock 62, 64, 93
*Empire and Sexuality: The British
    Experience* 80
End of Alice, The 133
Engels, Friedrich 58–9
Enlightenment 44–52
epigenetics 126
'erectile dysfunction' 110

erotic art
  Japanese 49
  'Mochica Pottery with Erotic Scene'
    17
  Pan sculpture 15–6
  Renaissance 26–7, 28
  Roman 15–6
erotica, as sexual sharing 24
erotomania 68–9
*Essential Prescriptions Worth a
  Thousand Pieces of Gold* 11
eugenics 60
Europe, early modern 23–7
evolutionary social theory 58
*Exposition of Cultivating the True
  Essence by the Great Immortal of
  the Purple Gold Splendour* 11

Family Planning Association (FPA) 89
family planning clinics 87, 88–90, 93
*Fanny Hill: or, the Memoirs of a Woman
  of Pleasure* 44–5, 132–3
female condom 91
female genital cosmetic surgery
  (FGSC) 113
female genital mutilation 67, 111–2
female orgasm 10, 56, 74, 98, 107–8
'female sexual dysfunctions' (FSDs)
  108–9
Femidom 91
Feminine Forever 86–7
feminism, work of Christine de Pizan 25
festivals 143
fetishism 65–7
films (list of) 138
Fire (film) 118–9
Flaubert, Gustave 37
Forster, E.M. 141
FORWARD (Foundation for
  Women's Health Research and
  Development) 110

Foucault, Michel 4, 22, 46, 57, 82, 128
free love 59–60, 103
Freud, Sigmund 4, 66, 98
Function of the Orgasm, The 95
*Functions and Disorders of the
  Reproductive Organs* 109

G-spot 30
Galen 18
Gandhi, Mahatma 142
Garrett Anderson, Elizabeth 69
Garfield, 141
Gauguin, Paul 37
gay movement 125
*Gay, Straight, and the Reason Why: The
  Science of Sexual Orientation* 127
Geneanthropeia 28, 29
genetic determinism 126–7
Gillard, Julia 102
Ginsberg, Allen 95
Gogh, Vincent Van 37
Goncourt brothers 74
Graaf, Reinier de 29–31
Greer, Germaine 105, 142
Griffith-Jones, Mervyn 100
Guislain, Joseph 66
Gynaecologia Historica-Medica 32
gynephilia 127

Haggard, Rider 83
Haire, Norman 86
Hall, Radclyffe 83, 132
Hall, Thomas/Thomasine 31
Hammond, W. A. 32
Haworth, Samuel 16, 18
Heliogabalus 15
hermaphroditism 12, 31, 78
Hijras 119, 141
History of Sexuality (Foucault) 4
Hite, Shere 99, 141
HIV 90–1, 106–7

Hokusai 49, 50
Homes, A. M. 133
homosexuality
  in Eastern culture (11th-15th cent.)
    27-8
  homophobia 122, 124
  as "illness" 122-4
  in the *Kama Sūtra* 12
  laws regarding 121-4
  origin of term 82
  pederasty 20, 79-83
  in Taoist writings 10
  Uranians 79-82
  see also catamites; lesbianism
Homosexuality in Perspective 99
Hooker, Evelyn 123
hormones 86, 109, 126-7
Hottentot Venus 62-3, *63*
Human Dignity Trust 122
human rights issues 101, 112, 120
Human Sexual Response 98
humoral theory 16
Humsafar Trust 119
Hyam, Ronald 80
hypersexuality 68-9
hysterization of women's bodies 57,
  70

'Imperfect Enjoyment, The' 40
impotence 110
'indeterminate' gender 120
India
  11th-15th cent. 27
  attitudes towards homosexuality
    118-9, 121
  hermaphroditism in ancient texts 12
  sexual laws 52
  see also Kama Sūtra of Vatsyayana,
insanity, eroticism leading to 18
International Lesbian, Gay, Bisexual,
  Trans & Intersex Association 120

internet pornography 114
internet sites 137
Ivonov, Eugene 134

Jacobi, Mary Putnam 69-70
Japan
  erotic art 49
  free love movement 59
Jarman, Derek 118, 125
Jefferson, Thomas 47
Johnson, Samuel 6, 48
Johnson, Virginia 98-9
Joyce, James 37

Kama Sūtra of of Vatsyayana, 11-3,
  78-9
Kapoor, Ranbir 119
Kathasaritsagara 27
Katsav, Moshe 135
Keeler, Christine 101, 134
Kerouac, Jack 95
Kertbeny, Károly M. 82
Khan, Imran 119
Kingsley, Charles 74-5
Kingsley, Fanny 74-5
Kinsey, Alfred 97-8
Kisch, Heinrich 108
kissing 99-100
Krafft-Ebing, Richard 55,
  63-4, 66, 69
Krittivasa Ramayana 27
Kunisada 49

L-Shaped Room, The 132
La Cazzaria (The Book of the Prick) 34
'La Chanson d'Audigier' 23-4
labiaplasty 113
*Ladder of Love – The Ascent to Beauty
  –Itself (Symposium)* (Plato) 18-9
Lady Chatterley's Lover 100-1
language of sex 34, 98-9

law
  Contagious Diseases Act (1860s) 38
  on homosexuality 121–4
  religious 26, 38–9
Lawrence, D. H. 100–1
'Le Chevalier qui faisoit parler les cons et les culs' 33
Le Petit, Claude 40
Le Sexe Qui Parle, (film) 33
Leda and the Swan 4–6
Leda and the Swan (Rubens) 6
Leda and the Swan (Yeats) 5
Lemnius, Levinus 51
Leonardo, da Vinci 26
Les Bijoux Indiscrets 33
Lesbian Sex Mafia 127
lesbianism
  during Enlightenment 48
  in Eastern culture (11th-15th cent.) 27–8
  less threatening than male homo-sexuality 83, 100
  in Taoist writings 10
LeVay, Simon 127
libido
  'normal'/'dysfunctional' 109–10
  women's loss of 108–9
Lister, Anne 83
Livermore, Mary 69
London Labour and the London Poor 61
Love Without Fear 99
Lullaby (Auden) 95–7
Lyon, Mary 126

McCarthy period 123
Magic Walking Stick, The 33
'Maiden Tribute of Modern Babylon' 52
Mailer, Norman 95
male circumcision 112–3
male menopause 109

Malinowsk, Bronislaw 93
Malleus Maleficarum ('The Hammer of Witches') 27
Malthus, Thomas 44
Marcuse, Max 44
Marie Stopes Clinic (Whitfield Street, London) 90
Marlowe, Christopher 14
marriage guidance 87
Marriage and Morals 88, 93
Married Love 87
masochism 64
Masters, William 98–9
masturbation
  childhood 51, 58
  female 10
  in public 71
Matthews, R. H. 61
Maupassant, Guy de 37
Mayhew, Henry 61
Mead, Margaret 85, 92, 98
medical discourse 28, 29–31, 44
Medieval Europe 23–7
Mehta, Deepa 118–9
menopause
  female 107–8
  male 109
menstrual blood 35
Messalina complex 68–9
Michelangelo 5, 28
Midwives Book 51
Miller, Henry 132
Milton, John 43
miscegenation 91
mistress, keeping a 48
Mugabe, Robert 122
Muggeridge, Malcolm 15
Munby, Arthur 76
music 133
Mysteries of Conjugal Love Reveal'd 31–2
mythology 20

Naked Lunch 133
Napoleonic Code 52, 80
National Association for Research
    & Therapy of Homosexuality
    (NARTH) 122–3
National Birth Control Association 89
National Survey of Sexual Attitudes
    and Lifestyle (NatSAL) 53
National Viewers' and Listeners'
    Association 114
necrophilia 66–7
Needham, Joseph 11
Neo-Confucianist puritans 11
NHS (Family Planning) Act (1967) 90
Nietzsche 37
Nin, Anaïs 132
'norms'
  developed by sexologists 98
  during Enlightenment 46–8
Noyes, John Humphrey 59–60
nymphomania 66, 68, 69

older people 106–10
On the organs of women which serve
    the purpose of procreation 29–31
'one-sex model' 18
120 Days of Sodom, The 3
Oneida Perfectionists 59–60
online porn addiction 114
oral sex 13, 16
orgasm, female 56, 74,
    98, 107–8
orgies 14–5
Origin of Species 58
original sin 22
Orlando: A Biography 133
Ovid 13–4

Paglia, Camille 20
Pan sculpture 15–6
'paraphilia' 65–7, 80

pathologizing sexual behaviours 56–8
pederasty 20, 79–83
  see also catamites
Perfumed Garden of Sensual Delight
    27–8, 79
perversion 58, 65–7, 80
Peter Pan 83
Petraeus, David 135
phallocentricity 110
physical attraction vs. spiritual
    loveliness 19
Picasso, Pablo 49
pill, the 90
Plato 12, 18–9, 80
plays (list of) 138
  see also Restoration Plays
pleasure, who has the most 20,
    30, 32
Poe, Edgar Allan 80
'Poetic Principle, The' 80
poetry 139
Polynesia, sexual
    attitudes in 47
popular culture 113–4
'pornodidascalian' works 28
pornography
  child 114
  first use of word 28–9, 56
  internet 114
  origin of word 39
  as 'sexual using' 24
Portnoy's Complaint 133
Prime of Miss Jean Brodie 141
printing press 27
Profumo affair 101, 134
promiscuity, 'base line' of 58
Psychopathia Sexualis 63–4
Puritanism
  backlash against 40–1
  'spiritual authority' of 38–9
Putin, Vladimir 121

qi (avoiding expending) 10
Queer Nation 125
Quensel, Nils 134
quotes 141–2
Quran 23

race
  different ages of consent 52
  other races over-sexed 58, 60–3
*Rare Verities, the Cabinet of Venus
    Unlock'd* 28
Reage, Pauline 132
Reed, Lou 5
Reich, Wilhelm 94–5, 102
Reid Banks, Lynne 132
rejuvenating treatments 86–7
religious law 26, 38–9
Restoration Libertines 40
Restoration plays 39–41
Rice-Davies, Mandy 101
Rochefoucauld, Count Gaston de la
    75–6
Rochester, John Wilmot, Earl of 40–1
Rodin, Auguste 49
Romans
  emperors' orgies 14–5
  erotic art of 15–6
  instructional texts 16
  Pan sculpture 15–6
Roth, Philip 133, 141
Rover, The 39
Rubens, Peter Paul 6
Rubyfruit Jungle 132
Russell, Bertrand 59, 88, 93
Russia 121–2
  see also Soviet Union

Sacher-Masoch, Leopold von 132
Sade, Marquis de 3, 49
sadism 64
Salinger, J. D. 95

salirophilia 76
Sanger, Margaret 93
satyriasis 68
Savonarola 141
Scharlieb, Mary 108
Schubert 37
Schurig, Martin 32
science *see* medical discourse;
    sexologists
*Secret Instructions of the Jade
    Chamber* 11
Secret Miracle of Nature 51
Secrets of the Alcove 44
Selwyn, George 66–7
sex addiction 68–9
sex scandals 101, 134
sex-change operations 94
sexologists 86–7, 97–100
Sexual Behaviour in the Human Female
    97–8
Sexual Behaviour in the Human Male
    97–8
sexual diseases 34–8
Sexual Inversion 64
*Sexual Life of Savages in North-
    Western Melanesia, The* 93
Sexual Life of Women, The 108
*Sexual Meaning of Procreation and
    Contraception* 44
Sexual Offences Act (1967) 124
sexual reassignment surgery 94
'sexual revolution' 40, 95, 102–3
sexual silence 4
sexuality
  ambiguity of concept 2–3
  definitions of 2
  origin of term 4
Shakespeare 141
Sharp, Jane 51
She 83
Shelley, Percy Bysshe 80

Simpson Miller, Portia 122
sin, link with sexuality 10, 22–3
Sinibaldi, Giovanni 6, 28
sodomy 45–6, 47
'Sotadic Zone' 82
Soviet Union 59
  see also Russia
Spark, Muriel 141
speculum 70
Spermatologia Historica-Medica 32
spiritual loveliness vs. physical
    attraction 19
State, dictates from the 4
Stead, W. T. 52
Steinach, Eugen 86
Steinbeck, John 1
Stevenson, Robert Louis 83
Stonewall 125
Stopes, Marie 87, 88, *89*, 93, 109
Story of O 132
Strauss-Kahn, Dominic 134
Studies in the Psychology of Sex 62
Sushruta Samhita 27
Symonds, John Addington 64, 81
syphilis 34–8

'Tako to Ama (The Dream of the
    Fisherman's Wife)' *50*
talking vaginas 32–3
Taoist writings (c.2000 bce) 10–1
'technology of the flesh' (Foucault) 22
testosterone 109
texts
  classic 140
  Roman instructional 16
  Taoist writings (c.2000 bce) 10–1
Thorpe, Jeremy 134
Tiberius 14–5
Todd, David 77–8
Todd, Mabel Loomis 77–8
Torella, Gaspar 35

Toulouse-Lautrec, Henri de 49
Transgender Europe (TGEU)
    119–20
transgender people 119–21
trial marriages 93
Tropic of Cancer 132
Twelve Caesars, The 14–5

Updike, John 132
Uranians 79–82
Utamaro 49

'Vagina Monologues, The' 33
Venette, Nicolas de 31–2
Venus in Furs 132
Viagra 109–10
Victoria, Queen 74
Victorian period 56–71, 74–83
Vignali, Antonio 34
violence, internet influenced 114
Voronoff, Serge 86

Walker, Alice 128
Wandering Whore 141
Ward, Steven 101, 134
Water Cherubs 81–2
websites 137
Well of Loneliness, The 83,
    132
West, Mae 141
Westphal, Carl 82
Whitehouse, Mary 114
Wilde, Oscar 37, 73, 83
Wilmot, John 37
Wilson, Robert 86–7
Winckelmann, Johann Joachim
    15
Winterson, Jeanette 128
witch-hunts 27
Wolfenden Report (1957) 124
Wollstonecraft, Mary 59

women
  hysterization of bodies 57, 70
  loss of libido 108–9
  older sexually active 107–8
  pathological sex-drive of 66, 68, 69
  as powerful corruptors 6, 24–5, 27
  for procreation only 29, 87–8
  sexual organs substandard 18
  social constraints (17th cent.) 39–40
  as transmitters of sexual diseases
    3, 35, *36*

weaker sex 16, 18
  see also female genital mutilation;
    female orgasm
Woodhull, Victoria 59
Woolf, Virginia 133

Yeats, W.B. 5, 86

Zappa, Frank 114–5
Zaretsky, Eli 103
Zuma, Jacob 135

ALL THAT MATTERS: SEXUALITY

All That Matters books are written by the world's leading experts, to introduce the most exciting and relevant areas of an important topic to students and general readers.

From Bioethics to Muhammad and Philosophy to Sustainability, the *All That Matters* series covers the most controversial and engaging topics from science, philosophy, history, religion and other fields. The authors are world-class academics or top public intellectuals, on a mission to bring the most interesting and challenging areas of their subject to new readers.

Each book contains a unique '100 Ideas' section, giving inspiration to readers whose interest has been piqued and who want to explore the subject further.